NATURAL REMEDIES FOR CHRONIC PAIN

A Comprehensive Guide

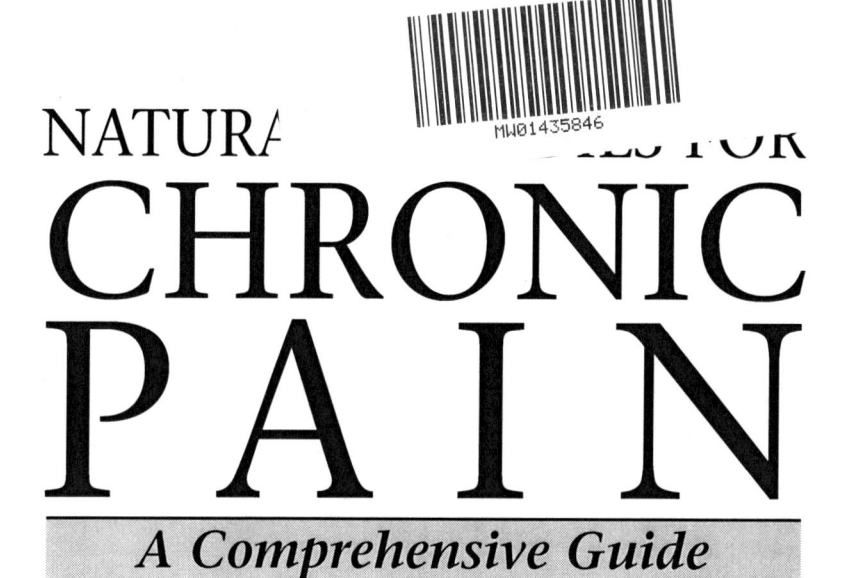

The Alternative Medicine Chronicles
VOLUME III

ROBERT SIBLERUD

New Science Publications
9435 Olsen Court
Wellington, Colorado 80549
(970) 568-7323
Rsiblerud@aol.com
www.Newsciencepublications.net

NATURAL REMEDIES for CHRONIC PAIN
A Comprehensive Guide

Copyright 2016
All Rights Reserved

Published by:
New Science Publications
9435 Olsen Court
Wellington, Colorado 80549

Printed in USA
ISBN: 978-0-9666856-9-5
Library of Congress Control Number:
2015918616

Acknowledgments:

Editing: **Margaret Shaw**
for the many years she has edited my books. Many thanks!

Proof Editor: **Shirley Parrish**

Inspiration for the Book: **Ron Irwin**
for his suggestion to write a pain book.

Cover Art and Layout:
Julie Melton, The Right Type Graphics

Other Alternative Medicine Chronicles:

**Mind Your Health, Heal Your Body:
A Guide to Wellness
Volume I**

**Cancer and Alternative Therapies:
A Comprehensive Guide
Volume II**

TABLE OF CONTENTS

Preface: Robert Siblerud iv

Chapter One
Understanding Pain: *Pain 101* 1

Chapter Two
Mind and Pain: *It May Be in Your Head* 19

Chapter Three
Mind as Healer: *Safer than Drugs* 29

Chapter Four
Back Pain: *Natural Remedies* 43

Chapter Five
The Illusion of Back Pain: *An Emotional Dis-ease* 61

Chapter Six
Arthritis Pain: *There May Be A Cure* 81

Chapter Seven
Fibromyalgia: *Pain and Fatigue* 105

Chapter Eight
Headaches: *It Is In Your Head* 129

Chapter Nine
Other Pain Disorders: *From Neuropathy to Feminine Pain* 139

Chapter Ten
Nutrition and Pain: *A Cause and Cure* 151

Chapter Eleven
Herbs and Nutrients for Pain: *From A to Z* 167

Chapter Twelve
Natural Therapies for Pain: *A Synopsis* 191

Appendix I: *Various Commercial Remedies* 219
Appendix II: *Making A Decision About Pain Therapy* 227
References and Suggested Reading 244
Index 247

PREFACE

If you are reading this book, you or a loved one are probably one of the 100 million American adults who suffer from chronic pain. That includes 40 percent of the population, according to a 2011 report from the Institute of Medicine. Confirming this study was a 2012 Gallup telephone poll of 353,000 American adults which found 47 percent of American adults suffered from some type of chronic pain. They found that between 10 to 30 percent of people with chronic pain hurt so badly, they are unable to function. These are astounding statistics. Before undertaking the research for this book, I had no idea that chronic pain was so prevalent. Many of the medical pain relievers are addictive, and even over the-counter-pain relievers can be deadly.

Several years ago Ron, a friend of mine, and I were sitting in the sauna at our condo complex. Ron, who has cancer, knew I was writing a book on alternative therapies for cancer, suggested I write a book about natural remedies for pain, because he was also suffering from pain. At that time I dismissed the idea but put it in the back of my mind. After finishing my cancer book entitled *Cancer and Alternative Therapies: A Comprehensive Guide*, I began to ponder the idea about writing a book about pain and natural therapies. I do have a high interest in pain. A number of years ago I received a sizeable grant to research light emission diode monochromatic light therapy for people with arthritic hand pain in cooperation with Poudre Valley Hospital in Fort Collins, Colorado.

After doing research for this book, I was surprised to find the number of good scientific studies conducted on natural remedies for pain. Most of these remedies are not being utilized by traditional medicine. Shortly before writing this preface I came across an excellent book, entitled *A Nation in Pain: Our Biggest Health Problem*, written by Judy Foreman. It contained the missing link to my book, explaining why much of the medical profession seems to be in the dark about treating pain. Pain is the primary reason that patients go to doctors.

Surprisingly, doctors are required to take only a few hours of pain education during their four years of medical school. Foreman writes that, "Most doctors know almost nothing about it." Wow! The National Institute of Health spends about one percent of its large budget on pain research, even though pain is a bigger problem than heart disease, cancer, and diabetes combined. Another amazing statistic is the risk of suicide for people with chronic pain, about twice as high as those without chronic pain, and even higher for those with severe chronic headaches. My grandfather, whom I never knew, committed suicide in 1923 because of severe chronic abdominal pain. The only way to relieve his pain was to puncture the abdomen to relieve the fluid build-up.

Foreman writes that the medical system does a "terrible job of educating doctors about pain." She states that 80 percent of medical schools don't teach pain biology and modern principles of pain relief, and palliative care is not taught to medical students." There are between 3,000 to 4,000 physicians who understand pain and are certified as pain specialists, but are unable to see the millions of people who suffer from chronic pain.

The burden of pain relief falls on the primary care physician who virtually gets no pain education at any point in their career. Dr. Mark Zylka, a University of North Carolina pain researcher states, "I teach a one-hour lecture on pain to medical students. That is about all they get." A survey by the American Association of Medical Colleges, which represents 135 accredited medical schools, found that medical schools taught on average 8 to 16 hours of pain education over four years of medical school. Another study found the median number of pain teaching hours was just 9 hours in the United States. In Canada it was 18 hours. Only four U.S. medical schools had a required course on pain, and a number of schools did not report any teaching of pain in their curriculum. A large number of schools devoted less than five hours to the pain topic according to a John Hopkins' study.

A 2001 national survey by Harvard Medical School found only half the doctors in primary care practice felt only 'somewhat prepared' to counsel patients about pain management. Another study found only 25 percent of graduates admitted their pain education was adequate. Dr. Joel Loesser, a neurosurgeon at the University of Washington stated, "The medical school curriculum is the last vestige of the feudal system in post-modern America. The curriculum is owned by the faculty of the school." In other words, they don't want to change.

The costs of chronic pain are enormous. It is the most common reason why patients go to doctors. It costs more than cancer, heart disease and diabetes combined. Pain accounts for about 42 percent of all visits to hospital emergency rooms. A 2011 study found chronic pain costs the United States between $560 to $635 billion a year in direct medical costs and lost production. Per capita pain costs range between $1,842 and $2,072 annually. A person with severe pain costs $3,210 more annually than a person with moderate chronic pain.

Statistics regarding mortality and pain medication should motivate sufferers to try natural remedies for pain. Every day, over 40 Americans die from abuse of prescription pain killers according to the Center for Disease Control (CDC). That totals over 15,000 people a year. Another 16,000 people die from over-the-counter NSAIDs, such as aspirin and ibuprofen. In other words, over 30,000 Americans die from pain medication annually. Yikes!

Overdose of opioid prescription drugs now kills more people in the United States than do overdoses from heroin and cocaine combined. Many people become addicted to narcotics during their pain therapy. One meta study analysis found that 3.3 percent of patients taking opioid prescriptions became addicted. A larger percentage will demonstrate drug related behavioral illicit drug use. The practice of taking pain killers, not for pain, but to get high has tripled since 1999. According to CDC director, Thomas Frieden, M.D., rogue doctors are a big part of the problem. A California study found 3 percent of doctors wrote 62 percent of pain killer prescriptions. Frieden emphasizes drug abuse problems originating from rogue doctors is much more than drug pushers on street corners. The drugs most abused are vicodin (hydrocodone), oxycontin (oxydodone), opana (oxymorphone), and methadone.

In 2010, pharmacies sold enough of these opiate-based prescription drugs to give every person in the United States a typical 5 mg of hydrocodone every four hours for one month. Narcotics should be the last resort for pain control. Prescription pain killers are now the leading cause in accidental deaths, over taking auto accidents. Dr. Frieden states, "We are in an epidemic of prescription drug overdose." There are safe solutions for chronic pain, and hopefully this book will enlighten pain sufferers about these safe alternatives.

Judy Foreman in her book asks why is there no Institute of Pain at the National Institute of Health. The government is doing almost nothing to address the chronic pain crisis. There is an advocacy group called Pain Action Alliance to Implement a National Strategy (PAAINS) formed to convince the government to do more regarding chronic pain. One suggestion is to require physicians to have more knowledge about pain by testing graduating medical students on their knowledge of pain. This would force medical schools to teach it, according to Dr. Scott Fishman, an anesthesiologist who heads the division of pain medicine at the University of California, Davis.

Evidence suggests that the medical profession is letting patients down regarding chronic pain. Patients need to be responsible for their own health. Remember that it may take up to a month before you see any relief when using some natural remedies. Hopefully, this book can be a guide that will lead to pain relief through natural remedies. It is always wise to consult with your health care practitioner when embarking on alternative therapies. Perhaps you can educate your doctor. Good luck with your journey!

Chapter One

Understanding Pain

Pain 101

You are about to discover the morbid world of chronic pain. Hopefully you are not one of the many millions of Americans who suffer from arthritis, back pain, fibromyalgia, headaches or 600 other forms of chronic pain. If you do, this book may give you hope to naturally cure yourself with natural remedies. Most pain sufferers seek relief from drugs and their multitude of side effects. Even the over-the-counter drugs, such as aspirin and ibuprofen cause over 16,000 deaths each year. Yikes! We will discuss in this chapter how the medical profession often seems to treat the pain symptoms with drugs and surgery and not treat the cause. Another discovery you will make is how much the mind is related to chronic pain. Anxiety, depression, insomnia, and stress all play a role in chronic pain. Besides mental problems, chronic pain affects work, relationships, activities, the family, and the pocketbook to name just a few of its ramifications.

The surprising fact that I discovered in my research is how many excellent studies have been conducted on alternative therapies regarding pain. Many of these therapies have been proven to be as affective as prescription drugs but are being totally ignored by mainstream medicine. Why? As we will discuss, big medicine is being controlled at all levels by big pharmacy. Natural remedies do not make the drug companies rich.

Big pharma controls congress, the FDA, medical schools, medical journals, hospitals, physicians, and the mass media. In Europe, drug companies are prohibited from advertising. Europe believes drug decisions should be made by the physician, not the consumer. Erectile dysfunction should be discussed in the doctor's office, not in the living room while watching the evening news with the kids.

The book will examine the causes of chronic pain, the mind body connections, various pain conditions, natural remedies, and innovative therapies. Most of these alternative therapies have undergone controlled scientific studies showing they are more effective than placebos. The placebo effect is a good example on how the mind can cure pain. About 25 percent of pain medication works by the placebo effect. It is the author's opinion that all disease, including chronic pain, originates in the mind at some level. This includes repressed emotions, anger, and stress that may be the source of one's pain. Before we explore alternative pain therapies, it is important that we understand some basic science underlying pain, the role of big medicine and pharmacology, and the incidence of pain in humanity.

Pain in Society

Pain is one of the major health problems in the world today. It is the number one symptom that brings a patient to the doctor's office. Pain has a dual nature. In many diseases, it is the symptom underlying the diagnosis. It is also a disease in its own right that needs relief and attention. Every chronic pain at one time began as an acute pain. The more severe the acute pain, the higher likelihood it may become chronic. In many cases depression, anxiety, or a catastrophic event is associated with the development of chronic pain after an injury or surgery. The International Association for the Study of Pain has classified 600 different pain syndromes. They also classify pain into three categories. Acute pain lasts less than one month. Subacute pain lasts from one to six months, and chronic pain lasts more than six months. Most practitioners categorize chronic pain as lasting more than three months. In many cases, chronic pain can persist for years.

The surprising finding in my research is just how many

people are affected by chronic pain. Studies have shown that 37 percent of the population in developed countries suffer from chronic pain, with 33 percent occurring in the United States. In developing countries, 41 percent suffer from this morbid condition while Nepal suffers the most at 47 percent. Ouch! Another study looked at adults who described their pain as moderate or severe, which comprised 25 percent of the adult population. An American study estimated that 10 percent of the adult population had severe disabling pain, while a British study found that 11 percent of the adult population who were pain free at the start of the year would develop an episode of pain lasting for three months during the year.

Surveys done in both developed and undeveloped countries found musculoskeletal pain, most notably back and joint pain, was the most dominant type of chronic pain. The majority of people suffering from chronic pain have multiple sites of pain. For example, chronic back pain will be accompanied by pain in other body sites.

Swedish researchers studied 14,000 people and found that only 30 percent of them consulted their physicians for pain, half of them with chronic pain, and two-thirds with musculoskeletal pain. In Italy, one third of visits to a physician involved pain. Both studies found 67 percent of the patients received a prescription for their discomfort. A U.S. study found 28 percent of adults who visited a physician in 2000 had musculoskeletal pain.

Chronic pain often peaks and plateaus during middle age. However, the prevalence of lower back pain continues to rise into old age as it does with those who develop osteoarthritis.

Pain differs with sex. Women report more persistent pain than men with greater intensity. They also have more pain-related disabilities. Women have more migraines, fibromyalgia, and temporal mandibular disorders, while men have more gout and cluster headaches. Both men and women suffer equally with back pain. In the United Kingdom, women are 1.4 times more likely to develop chronic pain. It is not understood why women have more pain.

Social economic conditions play a role in pain. Those who endure adverse socioeconomic conditions experience more pain that is more severe. A Canadian study found those living in areas of low income families suffered more arthritis compared to those living in higher income areas.

Children living in families whose parents have chronic pain are more likely to develop pain. It is surprising how many children do suffer from pain. One study found that 25 percent of children up to 18 suffered from chronic pain. In that study, males numbered 19.5 percent compared to 30.4 percent of females. Two studies examined the prevalence of chronic pain in the elderly, those 65 and older. One found that 50.2 percent of the elderly reported chronic pain and the other study reported 32.9 percent, with 23.7 percent of males affected and 40.6 percent of females.

Pain varies in different countries. A European study of 42,697 people found 23 percent of the subjects reported chronic neck and back pain. In Columbia, the rate was 9.7 percent compared to 42.2 percent in the Ukraine.

Pain in the United States is prevalent, disabling nearly 50 million Americans. Not everyone seeks medical help, with one study reporting 43 percent of people who experience pain actually seek help. The study found that 44 percent of pain sufferers treat pain themselves. For those who consult a physician, 88 percent have been to more than one physician for their pain.

Research has found that 75 percent of chronic pain sufferers have had to make lifestyle adjustments to cope with their condition. About 20 percent have taken a related disability leave from work and 17 percent of chronic pain sufferers have had to change jobs. About 13 percent require help with daily living activities. Over a third have missed work due to the pain. Mental health is also affected with nearly half of chronic pain patients experiencing depression. Ten percent have considered suicide.

Medical treatment does not always work. For those receiving pain medication, 70 percent report they still suffer from pain. About one fifth did not experience any pain reduction while 10 percent report their pain got worse. For those suffering from surgical pain, one study found half of them were under-treated.

Each year there are 500,000 knees being replaced by surgery and 230,000 hips. It is estimated that 67 million adults will have some form of arthritis by 2030. Arthritis is the most common cause of disability in the United States. Gary Null, Ph.D. writes in his book *Reverse Arthritis and Pain Naturally* that "currently accepted practices of treatment may actually be worsening your arthritis and causing other health challenges." A 2005 National Health Interview survey conducted by the Center for Disease Control found two thirds of the people with arthritis were under the age of 65, including 300,000 children. Null, who is a nutritionist, believes the high rates are due to one underlying cause, "excessive amounts of highly concentrated calories and few viable healthy nutrients." The inflammation agents that cause arthritis and other degenerative disease is the American diet, i.e. junk food, soft foods, hamburgers, French fries, hot dogs, etc. In other words, arthritis and degenerative disease that cause pain can be prevented and treated by lifestyle changes, which usually includes diet and exercise. The Center for Disease Control reports that 47 percent of U.S. adults with arthritis have at least one other serious disease or condition. Only one in four American adults engage in exercise, and as we will see later, exercise is important for prevention and treatment of chronic pain. The statistics are amazing regarding chronic pain, much of which could be prevented and treated with lifestyle changes and natural therapies. However, most pain sufferers will enter the traditional medical avenue of drugs and surgery. As we shall see, this avenue can be devastating and even deadly.

The Medical Establishment

Modern day medicine does not address the underlying cause of arthritis and many other lifestyle diseases. Their objective has been to save lives in the short term and not long term. Physicians use drugs and surgery to relieve pain and exclude natural remedies that could accomplish the same result. They don't treat the cause. Part of the blame has to lie with the patient who wants a 'magic pill' instead of changing their lifestyle, which may include diet and exercise.

A 1995 report by Millman and Robertson, Inc., documented that up to 60 percent of surgeries in the United States were unnecessary. An article in the *Washington Post,* August 2012, reported that health policy researchers at the University of Michigan studied cardiology procedures across the state and found 43 percent of the procedures should not have happened if the surgeons had followed medical guidelines. In 1980, 16 percent of surgical procedures were performed on an outpatient basis, that is, not in a hospital. By 2007, the number grew to 57 percent. Physicians who obtained ownership of Ambulatory Surgical Centers performed more surgeries after ownership. In 1996, there were 220 centers which grew to 5,360, with physicians owning 83 to 88 percent of them. A scientific consultant firm Exponent, Inc., estimated that knee replacement surgery would grow 673 percent from 500,000 to 3.48 million in 2030. Dr. Lucian L. Leape, a Harvard professor, analyzed and studied the medical profession. He discovered that American medicine was the number one cause of illness in this country. Before Dr. Leape, no one had analyzed published literature dealing with injuries and death caused by government protected medicine.

For over five years, Dr. Gary Null (who is often on Public Broadcasting System) and his staff compiled an enormous amount of research regarding the results of medical procedures. The findings were staggering. Their research found that the number one cause of death and injury every year was American medicine confirming Dr. Leape's study. Annually, nearly 800,000 people in the United States die and many more injured by the American medical system. Cause of death ranged from adverse drug reactions, improper transfusions, surgical injuries, wrong side surgery, etc. The study was confirmed by another independent researcher. Null discovered that a high percentage of medical procedures for many conditions had never been established by a long term double blind, placebo study on humans. How could all this happen in modern medicine?

His answer is the powerful pharmaceutical-industrial complex that has an enormous influence over all aspects of the health care system. By working with the insurance companies and for-profit hospitals, they utilize massive lobbying companies to control virtually all federal regulating agencies involved in health care policy including the Federal Drug Agency and National Institute of Health. They do this by placing their supporters, policy making physicians, and scientists into key regulatory positions. They control the medical school curriculum through lavish gifts and research grants. No one in the media is going to expose them because they fear losing their advertising revenue from big pharma. By controlling the media, they shape public opinion by funding front groups, foundations, and think tanks. Big pharmacy controls doctors and hospitals through extravagant gifts as do medical device companies. According to a September 30, 2014 report by the Centers for Medicare and Medicaid Services, in a five month period they lavished $3.5 billion of gifts to hospitals and doctors to entice them to use their products. Most of the contributions came in the form of cash payments, followed by in-kind gifts and services, travel expenses, and stock options. This sounds like corruption to me, but if not corruption, at least unethical.

Null's report was entitled *Death in Medicine*, which is considered to be "the most comprehensive review of the dark side of American medicine to date." The report was sent to 7,000 individuals including all members of Congress, all state legislatures, all governors, and 100 scientific journals. Not a single agency or journalist touched the issue.

In 2004, half of all Americans took one pharmaceutical drug, with one in six taking three or more drugs. For those over 65, five out of six took at least one medication. A recent report published in the *Journal of the American Medical Association* found prescription drugs taken as prescribed in hospitals was the fourth leading cause of death in the United States and Canada. They caused 106,000 deaths annually and over two million injuries in the United States. An estimated 90 percent of people suffering from chronic pain wind up being prescribed an opioid, despite little evidence that the drugs help much or are safe for long term use. Over-the-counter drugs such as aspirin and ibuprofen cause over 16,000 deaths per year in North America. Acetaminophen (Tylenol and generic) cause almost 80,000 people per year to be treated in emergency rooms annually because they have taken too much of it. The drug is the most common cause of liver failure in the country. Acetaminophen is the most common drug found in the United States, and is found as an ingredient in more than 600 over-the-counter and prescription medications, including allergy aids, cold remedies, fever reducers, pain relievers, and sleep aids.

The most popular pain relief drug is Vicodin, and in 2011 the prescriptions numbered 131 million. It contains an opiate called hydrocodon. Dr. Thomas Frieden, director of the Centers for

Disease Control stated that "accidental overdose from Vicodin and other pain relievers kills more people than car accidents in seventeen states." Vicodin and other drugs containing the narcotic hydrocodone are the most commonly prescribed medications in the U.S. Every day 46 people die from these drugs, or almost 17,000 people per year die from overdoses of the drugs. That is up more than 400 percent from 1999. Mixing pharmaceuticals can be a dangerous cocktail with unknown side effects. Drug manufacturers are not required to test drug combinations.

The FDA was founded to protect consumers and oversee the activities of big pharma. For decades it has been run by a board of directors comprised mainly of past and present CEOs and board members of multinational conglomerates it is meant to police. It is like the fox guarding the hen house. Dr. Null calls it a collusion in direct conflict with consumer interest.

There are an estimated 13,000 pharmaceutical drugs on the market. In actuality, only 50 percent of prescription drugs actually work for the person taking them. For example, 75 percent are ineffective for cancer patients. For depression, 62 percent are ineffective. The profits of the ten pharmacy companies in the Fortune Top 500 are greater than combined profits of the remaining 490 companies.

The China Study which involved Cornell University, Oxford University, and the Chinese Academy of Preventive Medicine surveyed diseases and lifestyle factors in rural China and Taiwan. The study found that people who ate the most animal based food developed the most chronic diseases. Those on a plant based diet were the most healthy and avoided chronic disease. Modern medicine tends to ignore nutritional causes of disease and alternative therapies that have been proven effective by science. Many sufferers from arthritis discover alternative therapies often when it is too late. Obesity is one of the major health threats today. Two-thirds of Americans are overweight and one-third obese. Obesity is 54 percent higher among people with arthritis.

The Institute of Medicine, which is part of the United States National Academy of Science refers to the nation's epidemic of medical errors. Even the FDA admits that "adverse drug reactions are one of the leading causes of morbidity and mortality in healthcare."

This high rate of mortality is confirmed by Dr. Gary Null's team of researchers in their publication entitled *Death by Medicine,* which concludes that the medical system causes more harm than good. That is quite a conclusion, but the statement is backed up with good data.

1. The number of people in the hospitals having adverse reactions to prescribed drugs each year total about 2.2 million.

2. The number of unnecessary and inappropriate antibiotics prescribed annually is approximately 45 million prescriptions.

3. The number of unnecessary medical and surgical procedures performed each year totals about 7.5 million.

4. The number of people unnecessarily hospitalized each year is 8.9 million.

Null's research found that the total number of deaths caused by conventional medicine is nearly 800,000 per year. Wow! The report concluded that the American medical system is the leading cause of deaths and injury in the United States compared to heart disease at 652,091 deaths in 2005 and cancer at 559,312 deaths. Studies estimate that 6.7 percent of hospitalized patients have a serious adverse reaction with a fatality rate of 0.32 percent. There are more than 2,216,000 serious adverse drug reactions in hospitalized patients causing over 106,000 deaths annually. When one takes antibiotics when they don't need them, it increases one's risk of getting infections later that resist antibiotic treatments. Only bacteria respond to antibiotics, not viruses. Many people with viral infections receive antibiotics. Deaths from hospital infections within 30 days after discharge was 99,000 in 2002 out of 1.7 million infections.

The following is a summary of mortality rates from medical errors.

Condition	Deaths
1. Hospital Adverse Drug Reaction	106,000
2. Hospital Medical Errors	98,000
3. Hospital Bed Sores	17,160
4. Hospital Infections	88,000
5. Nursing Home/ Malnutrition	4,630
6. Outpatient Adverse Drug Reactions	199,000
7. Unnecessary Surgical Procedures	37,136
8. Surgery Related	32,000
Total	581,926

A ten year death rate from medical intervention, according to Dr. Null's research, is 7,846,360 deaths! The mortality cost of medicine's errors exceed $215 billion a year. Perhaps it is time to look at alternative therapies which are safer and have fewer side effects.

Neurobiology of Pain

Now to the boring aspect of pain. How does it work? As we get along in the book, we discover that physicians often cannot explain why people have chronic pain. There is no physical cause to explain why their patient should be experiencing it. So the pain model needs to explain how this happens. So hang in there as we try to explain the science of pain.

Pain is often described in terms of sensory (ouch), affective (emotional), and cognitive (thinking). The sensory relates to the intensity, location, and quality of pain as served by the neural pathway called the nociceptive system. Nociception is the scientific term used to describe the process in which a noxious stimuli as they describe it, such as an injury, produces activity

Understanding Pain

in the sensory pathway that conveys painful information. Pain is like a fever, it is a symptom. Biologically, pain is a signal that the body has been injured. Then there is psychological pain, the emotional suffering. Accompanying this pain is behavior modification, the way a person reacts to pain and thinks about its meaning and possible remedy. Higher brain centers are involved with the perception of pain.

Chronic pain occurs when the pain mechanism goes awry or when certain diseases associated with pain become chronic. The symptom of pain itself then becomes a disease. With chronic pain lasting more than three months, there are multiple biological, psychological, and social consequences. Because of the stress caused by pain, people may suffer even more symptoms such as fatigue, muscle tension, insomnia, anxiety and depression and a vicious cycle can transpire. Chronic pain can either follow an injury or occur without a specific injury.

Nociceptors are tissue damage receptors. It is the brain, not the receptors, that produce the ultimate sensation of pain. For our purpose, we will refer to nociceptors as pain receptors. Pain originates from a stimulus acting upon a pain receptor. The nerves from the pain receptor serves as a pathway leading to the central nervous system. Three types of nerve fibers carry pain sensations to the dorsal root ganglion adjacent to the spinal cord. AB fibers conduct light pressure sensations and vibration signals. AO fibers conduct mechanical stimuli, sensations such as heavy pressure, squeezing, or tissue damage. The C fibers conduct heat and chemical sensations. These fibers lead to dorsal horn neurons near the spine that then project to the thalamus. The next part of the journey goes to a neural pathway leading to the somatosensory cortex in the brain. Here, information about the intensity and location of pain is registered. To account for the emotions of pain, another nerve pathway of dorsal horn neurons projects to the brainstem, then to the thalamus, and finally to the limbic system of the brain, which is the emotional center of the brain. Pain is only experienced when the thalamocortical (sensory) and the limbic (emotional) combine in the brain. This combination forms the subjective human experience.

The affective dimension of pain relates to emotion and feelings associated with pain such as distress, annoyance, and discomfort. This occurs in the limbic system of the brain. The cognitive dimension of pain relates to thoughts associated with pain. It involves analyzing the cause of pain and determining the most appropriate behavior to remove the pain. The frontal lobe of the cerebral cortex is involved with the cognitive dimension.

All parts of the body are covered with nerve endings that are programmed to respond to specific kinds of unpleasant sensations. A certain level of stimulus intensity has to occur before the nerve responds by sending a signal to the brain. There are twenty different types of stimuli for which there is a specific nerve ending programmed and ready to respond to pain.

Various types of pain exist. For example neuropathic pain occurs from nerve damage or dysfunction to any part of the body's periphery such as in the feet in diabetic neuropathy. Neuropathy pain includes phantom limb pain (after amputation), trigeminal neuralgia, post herpetic pain, and diabetic neuropathy. Sensations may include a burning or a shooting type of sensation. When peripheral nerves are damaged beyond the distal cell body, the nerve fiber initially degenerates. What follows is a clump of regenerated neuronal sprouts that form a neuroma but it fails to find their target. Spontaneous nerve activity occurs in the absence of a stimulus and pain occurs.

When cells are damaged through injury or disease, pain-producing substances accumulate in the fluid outside the cell. Some of these substances leak from the damaged cell, and some come from the lymph system. As a result, the blood vessels dilate to bring more blood to the area. This results in redness, heat, and swelling. This is inflammation. Pain-producing substances are activated and sensitize the neural pathway resulting in pain. The nerve fiber receptors detect these pain causing substances such as bradykinin. In other words, inflammation results from a normal immune response that increases the blood flow to the affected area such as joint pain in rheumatoid arthritis. Other substances (such as prostaglandins, leukotrines, noradrenaline, adenosine, ATP, and nitric oxide) sensitizes these nerve receptors (nociceptors) by lowering their threshold resulting in the receptor firing at lower intensity of stimuli. Nonsteroidal anti-inflammatory drugs (NSAID) such as ibuprofen and aspirin act peripherally to reduce the formation of prostaglandins and are the most common analgesic for inflammation pain.

Chronic pain is a pain lasting for a long period of time. There may not be any clearly identifiable cause. It may persist for many reasons such as ongoing tissue damage (nociception) such as advanced cancer, or persisting degenerative disease such as arthritis. In some cases the cause of chronic pain is difficult to identify. Some chronic pain may occur because of deficient norepinephrine in the neural pathway, while other chronic pain may be due to deficient serotonin in the pathway. Chronic back pain has been associated with reduced gray matter in the thalamocortical area of the brain, which may explain cognitive symptoms with chronic disorders such as forgetfulness and decreased ability to process information. There may be a genetic component to chronic pain combined with environmental factors such as increased number of life experiences of stressful or painful stimuli. If the pain stimulus persists, stress hormones such as cortisol, thyroid hormone, and human growth hormone are released to help fight the stressor. If the pain persists, the body is exposed to high concentrations of cortisol. Muscle wasting may occur, and the immune system may be suppressed.

The relationship between pain and injury is not always predictable and depends on the circumstances. Pain is a dynamic sensation generated by the nociceptors (pain receptors) that can alter its sensitivity according to need and circumstances. Acute pain follows tissue damage and persistent pain follows the apparent healing of an injury. Brief transient pain is sometimes called physiological pain. If tissue damage persists because of ongoing degenerative disease, activity in the neural pathway may also persist leading to chronic pain. Sometimes it does not revert back to the normal state even if the tissue heals, resulting in chronic pain.

Referred pain is pain felt at body sites that are remote from the site of tissue damage. For example, pain during a heart attack is felt in the left arm.

A normal non-pain neuron can make a chemical known as substance P. As a result, this activity in the neuron may lead to the perception of pain in the absence of a stimulus, due to gene activity. Another way persistent pain can occur without a stimulus is through the expression of sodium channels in the nerve. These are portals in the wall of the nerve cells which sodium passes to generate nerve impulses. Another method of pain transmission without a stimulus is by prolonged synaptic input that can generate long term or even permanent changes in these neurons which might account for chronic pain.

Body chemicals can also influence the nerve transmission. Compounds such as glycine, and peptides such as enkephalin and dynorphin, and nucleoside adenosine can all act to turn down the nerve receptor signal. Calcium also plays a role. It regulates the amount of a neurotransmitter sent from one pain nerve to the next in the dorsal horn ganglia of the spinal cord. Pathways of nerves coming down from the brain through the spinal cord function to modulate pain messages coming into the spinal cord. Substances such as serotonin and endorphins are involved in pain inhibition. Endorphins are the body's own natural opium messenger to reduce pain.

According to the 'gate theory' of pain, the duration and frequency of a nerve's message and its competition from other nerve signals plays a role in what information gets passed to the brain. Specific areas in the spinal cord are responsible for amplifying the pain message by releasing amino acids or the substance P, which expands the area of receptivity to incoming pain signals. The duration and frequency of a nerve message and the competition from other nerve signals play a role in what information gets through to the brain. The bodies of the nerve cells that transmit pain are located in the dorsal root ganglia, which are small specialized clumps of nerve tissue that run along the length of the spine close to the spinal cord.

Medical science has been found to be ignorant of most chronic pain syndromes. Certain conditions may cause chronic pain such as injury to a sensory nerve, chronic inflammation, muscle spasm, and central nervous disruptions which may all contribute to chronic pain.

This is probably more science than you wanted regarding pain but at least you can understand better why some people can have chronic pain without a physical cause. Inflammation is the main cause of pain and chronic disease. Inflammation underlies arthritis, heart disease, cancer, Alzheimer's disease, and many types of chronic pain. It is wise that we understand the inflammation process.

The Inflammation Process

"Every disease, every ache, and every pain revolves around inflammation," writes author Jack Challem in his book *The Inflammation Syndrome*. Inflammation, he writes "may be aggravated by physical injuries, frequent colds, flues, overweight, and eating the wrong types of food." Chronic inflammation breaks down our bodies that make us more susceptible to disease.

So what is inflammation? It is the body's immune system recognizing microbes or an injury as being foreign invaders and coordinating an attack to contain the damage. Inflammation causes the tiny blood vessels to dilate, which allows a variety of white blood cells to leak out and engulf the microorganism. If there is an injury, the white blood cells will engulf and destroy the damaged cells. This inflammation process signals the body to grow new cells and to contain the injury. Within several days, the inflammation process decreases and the body heals. However, in chronic inflammation, the inflammation does not go away. It can result in prolonged swelling, stiffness, redness, tenderness, and pain, which are inflammation's common symptoms. For most types of arthritis, these symptoms indicate inflammation. When blood vessels become inflamed, the risk of heart disease increases. For those with an inflamed stomach, the risk of ulcers increases. If inflammation is in the gastrointestinal tract, cancer may develop.

There are several blood tests that can monitor inflammation. One is called the 'sedimentation rate,' which indicates how fast the red blood cells settle and form a sediment. Inflammation causes the red blood cells to settle faster. However, a better indication of systemic inflammation is C Reactive Protein (CRP). High CRP levels are associated with a 4.5 times greater risk of suffering from a heart attack. Elevated CRP levels are also found in people with Alzheimer's disease, cancer, arthritis, diabetes, infections, and physical trauma.

The cause of inflammation is often related to a dietary imbalance or deficiency. A poor diet primes the immune system for a powerful and chronic inflammatory reaction. Inflammation triggers are the circumstances that precipitate a specific inflammatory response after the body has been set up for an over-reaction. One should avoid those conditions that could trigger inflammation. There are six categories which can trigger inflammation writes Jack Challem.

1. There is an *age related wear and tear* on the body that is associated with one's biological age. When tissue breaks down, the white blood cells are mobilized to clean up. The speed of the clean up is influenced by genetics, diet, frequency of infections, stress, and lifestyle. Key pro-inflammatory substances generally increase with age. One way to maintain a lower biological age is to reduce tissue breakdown and the inflammation it stimulates. Diets that are rich in vegetables and fruits contain large quantities of antioxidants such as vitamin C, carotenoids, and flavonoids. The antioxidants neutralize free radicals that cause tissue damage. Often people who eat a lot of foods rich in antioxidants look younger.

2. *Physical injuries* can accelerated the aging process. Specific injuries to the joints and muscles can initiate inflammation. Injuries often become the cause of painful and debilitating health problems such as arthritis.

3. *Infections* initiate inflammation. A January 2002 article in the journal *Circulation* reported that repeated infections greatly increase a person's risk of coronary heart disease. Repeated infections also maintain a higher activity of immune cells which can damage blood vessel walls. Vitamin E, vitamin C, and N-acetylcysteine supplements can reduce the inflammation symptoms of infection.

4. *Environmental stress* can cause inflammatory responses such as tobacco smoke, air pollution, and sunburn, all which can initiate both acute and chronic inflammation. Cold air can initiate a severe asthma attack. Asthma sufferers often have abnormally high levels of free radicals.

5. *Allergies and food sensitivities* are associated with inflammation. About 15 percent of North Americans suffer from seasonal rhinitis and millions more experience

non-allergic rhinitis. Many people are allergic to pollen from trees, grasses, and weeds. Food sensitivities are also allergies. Today many people are sensitive to gluten found in wheat.

6. *Dietary imbalances and deficiencies* can trigger inflammation. People who are overweight are at higher risk for osteoarthritis, heart disease, cancer, and diabetes. The type of fat cells that develop around the abdomen generates a large amount of inflammatory substances such as C Reactive Protein. In other words, obesity is an inflammatory disease. Many pro-inflammatory fats are found in cooking oils and packaged foods. Once a balance of dietary fats is restored in the diet, plus supplements, the body regains its natural ability to both turn off and turn on inflammation. Elevated blood sugar can increase inflammation in the body. People with insulin resistance often have high C Reactive Protein, associated with inflammation.

The key to reducing inflammation and thus chronic pain is diet, which will be discussed in a later chapter. However, the mind is closely associated with pain, and we will discover its role in chronic pain.

Chapter Two

Mind and Pain

It May All Be in Your Head

Your state of mind can influence pain. As you will discover in this chapter, the mind is one of the most important variables when it comes to pain. If the placebo pill (the mind) can alleviate pain in over 30 percent of the population, the mind can also cause pain. Repressed emotions from childhood traumas is at the root of most back pain and fibromyalgia. A high percentage of amputees still have pain in the amputated limb called 'the phantom limb' pain. Evidence will be presented how stress, depression, and anxiety all play a major role in pain. If the mind causes pain, it can also heal pain and that will be discussed in the next chapter. The mind is one of the most neglected aspects of health care, and some scientists believe it is at the root of most diseases. It affects the immune system, the healing process, and chronic pain.

Emotions

Art Brownstein, M.D. states in his book *Healing Back Pain Naturally* that "chronic pain almost always has emotional roots." Our emotions generate powerful chemical changes in the body, even if those emotions are repressed and one is completely unaware of the repressed experience. Painful or traumatic emotions that get repressed at an early age become stored in the body and create tension and stress writes Brownstein. Chronic pain is often a conditioned response to a deep-seated feeling of guilt or self-blame. When one feels guilty, the person unconsciously seeks punishment, and punishment always brings pain.

Emotional pain should always be shared and talked about so it can be released and healed. Dr. Bernie Siegal, in his work with cancer patients, learned that keeping in emotional pain is unhealthy, eventually leading to illness. By concealing emotional pain from others, one can create more pain in their life. By sharing pain, one relieves the body of its burden. Such pain may originate from a loss of a loved one, the pain of being lonely, or a loss of a job. By sharing your emotional pain, it can be physically healing. Emotions such as fear, anger, sadness, jealousy, disappointment, and resentment when suppressed and internalized can create a toxic chemistry, which leads to more pain. Thousands of studies have established the direct relationship between what we think and what manifests in our body.

Even Sigmund Freud suggested that pain was generated by the mind. He emphasized an association between pain and the mental processes of repression, aggression, and guilt. He proposed that pain could act as a punishment of the self. Freud believed pain could be seen as a means of communication of various emotions to others at an unconscious level, especially anger which is a call for help. Psychotherapist Thomas Szasz in the 1950s believed that pain could be an unconscious form of aggression towards others, and suffering could relieve guilt.

Pain researcher George Engel suggested that in the general population there are individuals who have a pain-prone personality. They had a family history of painful conditions, many were from lower socioeconomic status, and many had sexual maladjustments. Engel stated that a pain-prone patient was said to exhibit self punitive behavior, and actually experienced pain at times when he or she could have experienced pleasure. Psychological trauma at an early age is often associated with a greater likelihood of developing pain in adult life. This trauma includes both physical and sexual abuse. Both lay people and health professionals regard pain as either real or imaginary, meaning that it had physical origin or was a product of the mind and not real.

Pain can be experienced in the absence of disease or injury, and complaints may be out of proportion to any physical abnormality. It can be used as a means for expressing a variety of repressed emotions. The perception by pain sufferers when others regard their pain as imagined can create distress for sufferers. Whatever the cause, the pain is real for the sufferer.

Stress

Jill Baron, M.D., an integrative medicine physician believes that most illness begins in the mind, caused by stress. When the mind is under stress, the cells of the body do not function optimally. Dr. Hans Seyle, a 1972 Nobel laureate, is considered the father of the stress field. Seyle discovered that every time one thinks a negative thought, there is a negative biochemical reaction in the body. Cortisol, epinephrine, norepinephrine, catecholamines, and blood sugar are all affected. Low levels of anxiety and worry are examples of low level stressors. Stress can contribute to inflammation in muscles and joints, causing pain and arthritis. Angry, stressful, and negative thoughts all cause pro-inflammatory biochemical reactions in the body. According to the National Health Interview Survey, 75 percent of the population experience some kind of stress every two weeks. The National Institute of Mental Health estimates that 26 percent of Americans over 18 years suffer from a diagnosable mental disorder in a given year. Stress also leads to drinking, smoking, and overeating.

Margaret Caudill, M.D., Ph.D. in her book *Managing Pain Before It Manages You* states that chronic pain is a form of chronic stress. She writes "The mind and body are really one. They have never been separate and never should be viewed as separate." How you feel can influence your body's processes.

The change in your body that constitutes the flight-or-fight response is meant to be temporary to meet a challenge or threat. The heart rate increases, as does the breath rate and blood pressure, and blood flow to the muscles increases during chronic stress. The body can be extended beyond its capacity for reestablishing balance. Numerous symptoms may develop such as reduced immunity, sleep disturbances, fatigue, headache, poor concentration, increased muscle tension, anxiety, and depression. Dr. Caudill emphasizes that chronic pain fits the definition of adverse chronic stress. Chronic pain places physical stress on the body. The experience of pain can be increased or decreased by how you process your ability to cope with pain. One needs to balance the stress effect of the pain. This is why stress management can be very helpful in coping with chronic pain.

In Canada, a study identified stress as an important predictor for the development of back pain in both men and women. Most back injuries occur just preceding, during, or shortly after a major period of stress. The more stress, the more the nervous system is stimulated and the more the body is affected. Stress activates the sympathetic nervous system, which causes the muscles to automatically tense and tighten up. Long term stress experienced daily can damage the back by severe muscle tension, which can distort spinal alignment.

Many studies have shown that chronic pain is associated with high levels of life stresses. Patients with chronic pain report more recent adverse events compared to pain free controls. Stress is related to biological changes that can exacerbate the pain, such as vascular and ischemic pain conditions including angina, migraines, and Raynaud's condition.

The stress response, flight-or-fight, is caused by the release of adrenalin and other hormones such as cortisol and growth hormone. Fibromyalgia patients were found to have elevated evening levels of cortisol and lower 24 hour urinary free cortisol levels. There appears to be a dysfunction in the HPA axis (hypothalamus, pituitary, and adrenal axis). This alters the cytokine function, explaining enhanced inflammation activity. It appears the HPA dysfunction precedes the onset of symptoms. Stress leads to high cortisol (the stress hormone) levels secreted by the adrenal glands, which can lead to chronic disease and premature death. Cortisol is used as a biochemical marker of poorly controlled stress and pain. This is why it is so important for pain sufferers to undergo stress management to deal with their pain.

Anxiety

Along with stress comes anxiety, which is closely related to chronic pain. Often the anxiety precedes the pain but is definitely there for pain sufferers. Life is no longer normal for pain sufferers. Many will lose self worth, and often the anxiety leads to clinical depression. Many sufferers are unable to cope with the pain, which may lead to anger.

Fibromyalgia is closely associated with anxiety, depression, and chronic widespread pain. In 76 percent of fibromyalgia patients there is a co-morbid anxiety disorder. Anxiety disorders may include an obsessive disorder in 6.5 percent of fibromyalgia patients, social phobia in 19.4 percent, post traumatic stress disorder in 21 percent, and panic disorder in 29 percent. Pain is often a symptom of anxiety and depression. Co-morbid anxiety disorders are present in 35 percent of osteoarthritis patients and the same percentage in spinal pain disorders. Anxiety, depression, and psychological distress increase the risk and intensity of pain. This in turn increases distress giving rise to a vicious cycle.

Psychological tests, specifically the MMPI, given to chronic pain patients find them scoring higher in hypochondria, depression, and hysteria referred to as the neurotic triad. Neurotic individuals usually experience great anxiety. Closely associated with anxiety is depression, which contributes to this vicious cycle of pain.

Depression

There has been a great deal of debate in medicine about whether or not chronic pain is simply the physical manifestation of psychological trauma, depression, or hysteria. Dr. Caudill, M.D., Ph.D. believes the mind and body are intimately involved in the experience of pain. She writes, "in the absence of pain, feeling sad or worthless and having trouble sleeping or eating may lead to a diagnosis of depression. But in a person experiencing pain, these common symptoms can be indications of the struggle to live with pain." Depressed patients often complain of bodily aches and pain. In chronic pain, the pain does not go away with treatment of depression, although the pain experienced may improve.

In a United States study of 3,047 people out of a total of 10,371 major trauma sufferers found that 12 months after their injury, the pain was more likely to still exist if the patient had not been treated for the depression prior to the injury. Depression can predict the onset of new episodes of pain and can predict the risk factor for persistence of pain over an eight year period. Likewise, chronic pain also predicts the development of psychological distress. A study of elderly people found the treatment of depression alone significantly improved pain and pain related disabilities.

Pain can be a symptom of depression or anxiety. One study found that 70 percent of patients with depression reported only physical symptoms such as pain for their first visit to a physician. They did not mention depression. Another study found more than 50 percent of depressed subjects with chronic pain described only physical symptoms but no emotional complaints. Ten percent denied any psychological symptoms of depression. Pain should be treated on equal priority as depression. For patients with specific pain symptoms, 30 percent have a co-morbid depression disorder. Among men with chronic back pain and depression, 58 percent said the depression followed the pain. A survey of 716 patients with chronic pain found depression in 59 percent and anxiety in 56 percent. Both depression and anxiety predict an increased risk for chronic back pain. Depression also impedes the response to pain treatment.

A 1993 study of chronic back pain patients found 54 percent developed depression disorder before the onset of pain. Depression predated the onset of pain in 42 percent of patients in a 1990 study. Pain is widespread among depressed individuals in the absence of a pain related diagnosis. Another study found depressed patients reported more pain after abdominal surgery than non-depressed patients. Besides depression and anxiety, chronic pain is associated with disturbed sleep.

Sleep and Pain

The vast majority of patients with chronic pain suffer from sleep disorders, especially initiating and maintaining sleep. Pain disorders often associated with sleep difficulty include fibromyalgia, headaches, oro-facial pain, and pelvic pain. Chronic pain patients with sleep disruption report more severe pain, pain of longer duration, greater disability, and more emotional distress. Both anxiety and depression are associated with insomnia, and the pain related symptoms could be underlying the cause of both. Patients whose sleep improved after insomnia treatment reported reduced emotional distress and pain related disability.

Medical experts state one of the best ways to reduce pain is to get sufficient sleep. Some people who wear stretch gloves, hose, and body stockings while sleeping have less pain and swelling, and thus sleep better.

Fatigue refers to decreased energy and feelings of being tired. Studies show pain causes fatigue. Chronic pain sufferers say they could stand their pain much better if only they could get a good nights sleep. They never feel rested and feel their resistance is weakened by lack of sleep. Often they feel worn out and exhausted with chronic fatigue. Frequently these sleep deprived individuals become irritable with family and friends, resulting in fewer friendships and fewer interests because of their preoccupation with pain.

Fibromyalgia patients spend significantly more time awake in bed and have a significant reduction of deep and REM sleep. This can lead to mood disorders, musculoskeletal symptoms, and even psychotic symptoms.

Valerian is a pink flower that grows wild in Europe, Asia, and America and has been used for centuries to treat insomnia and anxiety. Studies have shown it does help for sleep and does not lead to addiction with no known side effects. In Europe, it is widely used as a sedative.

Anger

Research has shown anger is associated with chronic pain. Anger is a negative emotion elicited by a perceived wrong. It is a transient state, while hostility refers to an enduring tendency to interpret others' behavior as malicious and aggressive. Hostile individuals are likely to be aggressive and often cynical. Aggression refers to the behavior component of anger. Controlled studies have shown higher levels of anger in patients with chronic pain compared to pain free individuals.

Anger is associated with greater pain and a higher level of psychological disturbances. Studies have shown those scoring high hostility scores with high anger expression scores in anger evaluation tests, can predict the highest pain levels among men. High hostility with low anger expression scores predicted the greatest pain among women.

Anger has been widely observed in chronic pain patients.

One study found 'bottled up' anger occurred in 53 percent of chronic pain patients. If pain persists beyond two to four months, depression, distress, and anger often develop.

Childhood Abuse

Many studies provide evidence regarding an association between chronic pain and a history of childhood sexual or physical abuse. Rates of self-reported sexual or physical abuse in patients with chronic pain range from 28 to 48 percent. Stressful, traumatic, and abusive experiences during childhood predispose individuals to develop chronic pain as an adult. A survey conducted on 91 patients with chronic pain found childhood abuse in 55 percent, with physical abuse occurring in 37 percent and sexual abuse in 27 percent. Another study found that sexual abuse increased the risk for arthritis in women, and physical abuse in childhood increased the risks for headaches. A study involving 90 females with chronic pain found nearly half had childhood abuse, sexual abuse in 18 percent and physical abuse in 11 percent. A high frequency of self-reported abuse were also found in chronic pain syndromes such as fibromyalgia. Those who were abused have poorer related adjustments to their pain.

A very interesting finding shows up between self-reported abuse subjects and those whose abuse is documented. The documented abuse subjects were no more likely to report pain than subjects without a pain history. Those subjects who retrospectively reported a history of abuse or neglect were more likely to report pain compared to a control who had no abuse history. Perhaps the retrospective self-report group repressed the emotions of abuse that later manifested as pain.

Childhood trauma may produce enhanced pain sensitivity. Studies by George Engel found those who were prone to pain had certain childhood occurrences that could account for their chronic pain. They include:

1. Physically or verbally abusive parents.
2. Harsh or punitive parents who over compensated with rare displays of affection.
3. Cold or emotionally distant parents who were warm when the child was ill.
4. A parent who suffered from chronic illness or pain.

Mind and Pain

Engel emphasized there was no single personality type predisposed to pain-proness but many types. He did find that most chronic pain sufferers repressed early trauma experiences. He found they suppressed guilt and anger that formed the foundation to vulnerability and suffering later in life.

A retrospective study found early trauma as described by Engel may predispose an individual to the development of low back pain. Personality disorders typically begin in adolescence and continue through adulthood. This reflects a long standing pattern of poor adaptation to life and its stresses. These disorders appear to be quite common among chronic pain patients. Between 18 to 59 percent of chronic pain patients have a personality disorder diagnosis. When chronic pain occurs in one of these disorders, treatment approaches are unlikely to be very effective. Early developmental trauma and the personality traits that are associated with it provide a vulnerability to pain and suffering.

An early traumatic experience such as loss or abandonment lays a foundation to pain-proness and psychic suffering. In many cases this matrix of unconscious factors lies dormant encapsulating the consequences of early childhood trauma until life events later trigger the repressed emotion. The life event may include a physical or psychic trauma or an illness, writes Robert Gatchel in *Psychological Approaches to Pain*. This trigger provides a theater for expression of the long-hidden conflict which plays out as chronic pain and the suffering that accompanies it. Gatchel states that in clinical work with chronic pain patients, it is often the suffering, not the pain that poses the primary problem. The chronic pain syndrome consists of both pain and suffering. Many patients express their pain and the suffering it causes as punishment for a past transgression. Some individuals can identify the event for which they believe they are being punished and others cannot.

Freud believed the most common of painful conditions are those which are chosen for hysterical conversion. The pain is very real, divorced from their physical origin. Pain that continues long after tissue has healed is a frequent occurrence. Chronic pain often reflects the psycho-dynamic issues that prolong clinical symptoms. This encapsulate a previous conflict, which is repressed that would otherwise reach awareness and cause anxiety.

Chronic pain patients do not come to pain management clinics for psychotherapy but for pain relief. However, the patient must be educated about the importance of psychological factors of the pain experience. A substantial percentage of chronic pain patients have a psychiatric disorder which should be evaluated. When the chronic pain syndrome occurs together with a psychiatric disorder, it is necessary to treat concurrently the disorder for any lasting relief from chronic pain. Often chronic pain patients resist being told their pain is associated with psychological problems originating from repressed childhood emotions.

Ergo Mania

Another cause of chronic pain can be found in the workplace called ergo mania. Ergo mania is a conflicted work ethic that may be an important characteristic of many chronic pain patients. These patients have a history of excessive work performance, relentless activity, self-sacrifice, and a precocious assumption of adult responsibilities writes Robert Gatchel. Ergo mania was one of only two psychological variables associated with pain. The other is repressed emotions. Studies have found patients with chronic pain compared to a control group have a great deal of ergo mania.

Phantom Limb Pain

Between 50 to 80 percent of amputees experience pain in the amputated limb long after the amputation. Those with a congenital missing limb do not experience it. Most often it occurs in the arms than legs. There is no evidence there are psychological factors involved.

Phantom limb pain illustrates the mind-body connection of pain. Years after individuals have lost a limb they are still experiencing pain as if the limb still existed.

As we shall discuss in the next chapter, the mind can also heal pain.

Chapter Three

Mind as Healer
Safer than Drugs

We have seen how powerful the mind is in causing chronic pain. If the mind can cause pain, the mind can heal pain. There are many techniques that can be used by the mind to relieve pain. They include biofeedback, relaxation techniques, coping skills, cognitive therapy, hypnosis, visualization strategies, and prayer to name a few. All have been shown scientifically to reduce pain. The best evidence of the relationship between the mind and pain is the placebo effect.

The Placebo

The placebo effect is one of the best examples of how the mind can control disease and pain. For decades during the last century, the placebo had been used as a standard therapy, but today it is rarely used. In the author's opinion, it should be used more often with pain. One can easily switch to a prescription drug if it does not work. The placebo works over 25 percent of the time for pain as demonstrated in studies where it is used as a control. Placebos have also been effective in improving function and stiffness in pain patients. Factors that influence the placebo effect include the patient and practitioner's expectation of improvement, relief of anxiety, and the patient doctor interaction.

The double-blind controlled study was developed to eliminate bias of both the researcher and subject. In other words, the studies are controlled against the placebo effect. Placebos can actually be more powerful than potent active drugs. Some patients can become addicted to placebos, and when discontinued, they can suffer withdrawal symptoms. Placebos have routinely been used for physical symptoms but now have been used effectively for psychological symptoms. Positive placebo effects are reported more frequently in patients with anxiety and depression. Hope and faith are important variables. Suggestibility appears to increase with stress. However, modern medicine no longer relies on the placebo effect.

Potent analgesics like morphine relieve pain in 65 percent of patients. Yet 25 percent of these patients may experience pain relief irrespective of whether they are given morphine or a placebo. The other 35 percent do not respond to either morphine or the placebo.

Studies have shown that placebos increase pain tolerance. Placebo tolerance was found more in anxious subjects compared to non-anxious individuals. Some researchers believe the placebo analgesic for severe pain may be a result of the patient's chronic anxiety level.

A 1974 double-blind study found that 36 percent of 908 patients were able to achieve 50 percent pain relief from placebos. Another study demonstrated 33 percent of pain patients experienced pain relief. A 1959 meta analysis of 15 studies revealed 35 percent of 1,082 pain patients had relief from a placebo.

People who respond better to placebos have a personality that is more expansive, cooperative, and uncomplaining, and are regular church goers, and have less formal education. Patients who were anxious and depressed also respond better to placebos. Blacks are more responsive to placebos compared to Caucasians.

Placebos are believed to stimulate opiate receptors in the brain. A 1978 study by Levine and colleagues demonstrated placebo-induced analgesics are mediated by the endorphin mechanism. It is reversed by an injection of Naloxone, an opiate antagonist. It would seem to be common sense to use placebos in pain management instead of harmful narcotics. Patients could be told there would be no side effects.

Biofeedback

Biofeedback is widely accepted by the medical community as an effective tool in reducing pain. It uses electronic instruments to measure body functions and then feeds the information back so one can learn to control the body functions with their mind. For example, fibromyalgia patients can learn to relax tense muscles to ease pain. Raynaud disease is a little understood condition in which the fingers and toes show an exaggerated sensitivity to cold. The cause is unknown. Raynaud patients can increase circulation and raise their hand temperature to relieve pain. Biofeedback helps people to become aware and then to control a specific part of the body and its function. All this is done with the mind. Research has shown that properly trained people can use biofeedback to relieve chronic pain, stress, anxiety, muscle tension, and gastrointestinal disturbances.

During a biofeedback session, sensors are attached to the part of the body being monitored. The sensor is connected to an electrical instrument, most often a computer. The biofeedback practitioner will instruct the subject in some mind-body techniques such as visualization or relaxation to influence the subconscious (autonomic) body processes. The instrument then feeds back on how one's thoughts are effecting the body by way of sound, light, or other signals. With practice, subjects learn what mental techniques to use in order to achieve the desired physical effects. Biofeedback has been shown to improve function and to relieve pain and stress for a number of conditions, especially when combined with relaxation techniques.

A controlled study of patients with rheumatoid arthritis found biofeedback and relaxation provided significant improvement in pain, tension, and sleep patterns when compared to physical therapy. Another biofeedback study when combined with behavioral therapies on rheumatoid arthritis patients found reduced clinic visits, hospital days, and lower medical costs over 18 months. Several studies have shown biofeedback helped patients with Raynaud's syndrome by teaching them to raise hand temperature and increase blood circulation.

One of the most common uses of biofeedback has been in the treatment of chronic headaches. The goal is to reduce muscle activity in the forehead muscles and/or increase skin temperature.

Studies have shown biofeedback can improve approximately 40 to 50 percent of tension and migraine headaches, comparable to drug therapy. Studies have also shown it to be effective for temporal mandibular disorders and back pain. Biofeedback is very beneficial for treating chronic pain, especially when combined with other treatment approaches. Other conditions helped by biofeedback include asthma, anxiety, attention deficit disorders, epileptic seizures, insomnia, substance abuse, and pelvic pain.

There are no side effects with biofeedback. Thousands of biofeedback practitioners are certified by the Biofeedback Certification Institute of America that can supply referrals.

Relaxation Therapy

Relaxation therapy is a systemic approach to train people to gain awareness of their physiological responses in order to acquire both a mental and physical sense of tranquility without the machinery of biofeedback. It rids the body of stress, anxiety, and tension. When muscles relax, they lengthen and allow the capillaries in the muscles to open. This reduces inflammation and pain. When both the mind and body are relaxed, stress is released and healing occurs.

The major forms of relaxation include breathing, guided imagery, progressive muscle relaxation therapy, meditation, and autogenic training. Through relaxation therapy, the patient learns how to decrease the amount of tension in areas of the body. There are fourteen muscle groups that can be relaxed during relaxation therapy such as upper arms and thighs. Relaxation therapies include:

1. *Breathing:* Breath is the link between mind and body. When a person is anxious or under stress, the breathing is disturbed. Improved breathing provides increased oxygenation to the body.

The key to relaxation is focused awareness. Breathing can be the object of that purpose. By focusing on how you breathe may provide you with an additional tool of relaxing. There are two types of breathing. Chest breathing is when you suck in the abdomen and express the chest with each breath. People who have prolonged anxiety are chest breathers. Stress increases the tension of the abdomen. Diaphragmatic breathing is when the abdomen rises and falls. Everyone starts as a diaphragm breather but then become chest breathers. A diaphragmatic breath is fuller and complete and can bring a feeling of calm and relaxation when it is done purposefully. There are diaphragmatic breathing exercises. Focusing on the present moment will allow you to consider what is upsetting you. When one first learns relaxation therapy, relaxation tapes can be very valuable. Use a focus word or phrase that keeps the mind in focus.

Proper breathing is a slow, controlled rhythm and is the fastest pain reliever you can use writes Vijay Vad, M.D., in his book *Arthritis RX*. It shifts the muscle attention away from the pain and to the body's natural response to pain. Breathing techniques are key factors of many relaxation and stress reduction techniques.

2. *Imagination:* The next step is to couple breathing with imagination. Imagine the breath going to areas of tension such as face, neck, back, or hand. One can imagine the breath coming in through the right hand and leaving the left hand.

Another imagination technique is to relax and imagine one's self in the environment that is safe, pleasant, and incompatible with the pain. For example, imagine lying on the beach. Guided imagery by a therapist can take the subject to an inner journey of serenity and peaceful places. One can also self-guide this journey.

The brain always converts these images, real or imagined, into electrical impulses before transmitting them to the body through the nervous system. One can worry and develop an ulcer. One can use imagery to heal back pain. The mind has incredible power to control pain and heal the body. If someone feels a headache coming on, he or she could imagine being in a beautiful mountain retreat listening to singing birds. Guided imagery is a legitimate form of relaxation therapy to help reduce pain or eliminate it all together.

Imagery is frequently used in treating chronic pain, cancer pain, tension headaches, migraines, stress, and anxiety. Studies have shown postoperative imagery provides less pain and lower dosage of pain relief drugs. A study on 58 fibromyalgia patients found it significantly reduced their pain and anxiety. Other studies have found imagery to relieve lower back pain and pain in osteoarthritis patients.

3. *Progressive Muscle Relaxation:* This technique involves alternatively relaxing and tensing various parts of the body, called progressive muscle relaxation. For example, curl the toes of the right foot on the 'in' breath and relax them on the 'out' breath. The purpose is to isolate each muscle group systemically by practicing tensing and relaxing various groups of muscles.

The process is to create tension for 8 to 10 seconds and then relax the muscles and let the tension release. Relaxed muscles require less oxygen so the breathing should be slow and deep.

4. *Autogenic Training:* The term autogenic means generated from within. The premise is that the body should follow the dictate of the mind. For example, say 'my hand is warm' and try to believe it. Research has found that autogenic relaxation is effective for insomnia, headaches, and chronic pain.

Autogenic training refers to a series of mental exercises and auto suggestions that are practiced regularly. The purpose is to have the individual switch off the stress response at will. The resulting passive state is thought to allow the brain and body to tap into its own spontaneous self-regulation mechanism. Autogenic refers to any method that patients use their own resource to help themselves heal. In a clinical setting, it is used to treat headaches. Controlled studies found autogenic training is helpful with hypertension, asthma, intestinal disorders, glaucoma, and eczema. It is useful in chronic pain. One controlled study found it useful as an adjunct therapy for complex regional pain. In summary, autogenic training is a meditational form of relaxation focused on very specific instructions.

5. *Environmental:* In order for these relaxation techniques to work, the patient should be in a safe, calm, and comfortable environment. This is essential for success. There

should be no disturbance. For a person in a high state of anxiety and distress, a calm environment makes it much easier to relax.

Cognitive Behavioral Therapy (CBT)

CBT is the most commonly used and scientifically valid form of psychological treatment and management of pain. The underlying premise is based on the assumption that thoughts and environmental events influence the experience of pain and a patient's response to pain. By intervention to alter thoughts and environmental situations, psychotherapists find it a very effective component of pain management. Treatment helps remedy the negative thinking pattern. Thoughts can influence emotional and physiological responses, which in turn influence behavior. Behavior is also influenced by environmental events. If patients are to learn effective techniques to cope with pain, they must also be an active participant in treatment. CBT involves relaxation training, education, pleasant activity, restructuring attitudes and thoughts, and pacing activities to reduce stress. Cognitive behavioral therapies include:

1. *Coping:* Coping is how the individual responds to their pain. A standardized evaluation, Coping Strategies Questionnaire, can assess a person's ability to cope. Pain coping can predict pain severity and how pain interferes with activity. Coping skills are an important predictor of a successful pain management program. Good coping skills can increase pain tolerance. Current pain management programs now emphasize coping more than the cure of pain.

Studies have shown that a patient's attitude, beliefs, expectations about their pain and themselves, and their coping skills affect their response to pain treatment. Coping is regarded as the effort an individual makes to manage and minimize the negative experience of pain. Coping strategies help change beliefs that individuals have about their degree of pain control. Without effective coping skills, one is likely to feel helpless and hopeless.

2. *Self Efficacy:* The self-efficacy theory states that change, whether behavioral or mental, relates to a person's belief about their ability to gain mastery over their pain. Mastering pain is the primary objective. Increasing self efficacy occurs through the process of improving coping strategy. One study found that cognitive strategy increases perceived self-efficacy and ability of the patient to endure and alleviate pain.

Self-efficacy refers to the belief in oneself that he or she can accomplish an outcome through one's own efforts. In lab settings, an individual's belief in their ability to tolerate pain can predict their actual response. College students who suffered from persistent pain had lower self efficacy scores compared to pain-free individuals. Self-efficacy is an important indicator of pain related symptoms. In a study of subjects with knee osteoarthritis, high self-efficacy levels were associated with better functional outcomes over a three-year period. In other words, self-efficacy protects against functional declines.

Enhancing self-efficacy should be a vital goal for treatment. Self-efficacy can be increased by various methods that include:

    I. Enacting a behavioral treatment program that involves performing activities that they may not otherwise engage in, according to Roger Fillingim, Ph.D., in his book *Concise Encyclopedia of Pain Psychology*. An example might be a supervised fitness program.

    II. Self-efficacy can be enhanced through vicarious experiences such as group treatment and observing coping skills of others.

    III. Self-efficacy can be improved through verbal persuasion by a good therapist.

3. *Attitudes:* The mind is the source of all thoughts, and feelings give meaning to the experience of pain. A self-defeated, hopeless mind set will probably contribute to the interpretation of pain in a negative way, such as distress and despair. The mind can be viewed as a filter though which the pain signal passes and is either magnified or dampened in intensity.

A person has no control over an actual event. It is how one reacts to the event that can affect health. A person always has the freedom to choose how to perceive an event, either positively or negatively. One has the choice of being angry and blaming another, and that response will create unhappiness. Anger has been widely observed in individuals with chronic pain. Chronic patients perceive a lack of control, which relates to their ongoing but unsuccessful effort to control pain. Their control has been taken away. However, one could perceive the negative event with a positive attitude and see the 'silver lining.' This could prevent a lot of anxiety by turning a negative situation into a positive situation. It is one's attitude that determines the response. Many studies have shown numerous health benefits for those people who shed rigid, destructive behavior, and negative thoughts, and who adopt a positive attitude with more flexibility. Studies show a positive attitude will decrease the risk of heart attacks and will increase the life span of cancer patients.

Many patients with chronic pain assume an attitude of helplessness. Often they hold feelings of blame and anger. Depression and anxiety, hallmark symptoms of chronic pain, underlie anger. Often there may be a forgiveness issue underlying chronic pain. The individual has a choice to harbor the negative feelings or forgive. Letting go of negative feelings will liberate both the mind and spirit.

Optimism is a healthy attitude. Optimists anticipate the best outcome that has been associated with an enhanced immune system. Optimism has been associated with the length of cancer, the more positive attitude, the longer the remission. Pessimism has been associated with depression and poor health. We always have the choice on how we view a negative event, either positively or negatively, with the latter being bad for health. A landmark book to read is *The Power of Positive Thinking* written by Norman Vincent Peale, which gives principles on developing a positive attitude. It has helped millions. Affirmations are one way to change attitudes, affirming oneself to look at the positive in all circumstances. A positive attitude will give one better self-esteem, which is diminished with chronic pain.

Humor is an important tool in remedying a negative attitude. It is important to be able to laugh spontaneously, which aids in optimism and a positive attitude. Norman Cousins wrote a book entitled *Anatomy of an Illness* describing how he cured himself of a mortal disease by laughing. He did it by watching funny movies and sitcom reruns. Laughter stimulates the production of endorphins and encephalins, both of which reduce pain. They are more powerful than heroin or morphine in modifying the pain response. Exercise also stimulates these two hormones. When one is laughing and enjoying oneself, the mind is at complete ease. The beneficial biochemicals released into the blood stream by humor help the healing process.

Prayer and Spirituality

Most Americans have a religious and spiritual background. Studies have shown that 75 percent of Americans pray regularly, and 79 percent believe that faith helps people recover from illness. Several studies have shown that prayer is one of the most commonly used alternative therapies for arthritis and is often rated as being the most helpful. Ironically, health professionals rarely mention religion and spirituality in relationship to health. Nearly 300 years ago during the scientific revolution, the practice of medicine separated from religion.

Spirituality is a personal search for meaning or connection with a higher power. Religion refers to an institution with established rituals and beliefs shared by others. Several studies have shown people who attend religious services take better care of their health. One study of 5,286 people over 28 years found frequent attenders of religious services had a lower mortality rate and were more likely to stop smoking, increase exercise, increase social contact, and stay married. A five-year study of 1,931 people who attended religious service had a 24 percent lower mortality rate compared to those who did not. There are many good studies that have shown the power of prayer in healing.

Art Brownstein, M.D., in his book *Healing Back Pain Naturally* listed some spiritual principles that can heal pain which include:

1. Avoid blaming yourself or others for your pain.

2. Don't live in fear and don't be afraid of pain.

3. Honor you pain as a teacher and friend.

4. Share your pain. You will heal faster if you talk about it.
5. Learn to love your body where the pain is located.
6. Learn to love yourself because love is the greatest healing force in the universe.
7. Develop healthy and loving relationships, which will help with one's pain.
8. Develop a sense of sense of unity and harmony.
9. Develop empathy with others and give up judgment.
10. Learn to acknowledge a higher power in your life.
11. Develop a gratitude for natural abundance in your life.
12. Practice forgiveness.

One study discovered that over time, the increased practice of praying or hoping was associated with decreased pain. All this is related to a positive attitude.

Meditation

Meditation has been very well studied showing that regular meditation can profoundly affect the physical body. Research has shown it can significantly relieve chronic pain and anxiety. A 1993 study on 77 fibromyalgia patients, who meditated for 10 weeks, found all 77 showed improvement and 51 percent showed moderate to marked improvement. A University of Massachusetts Medical Center study revealed chronic pain patients who had not improved with conventional medicine care, found half of them showed 50 percent improvement following ten weeks of meditation. Another controlled study found 60 percent of 225 meditators with chronic pain continued to show improvement four years after the study. Research of 28 women with fibromyalgia who meditated for eight weeks and who also practiced qigong, a Chinese exercise program, with pain management techniques had significant improvement in pain threshold, depression, coping, and functioning. The effects lasted four months.

Meditation promotes healing, calms the mind, promotes mental tranquility, soothes and relaxes the nervous system, and reduces muscle tension of the back. Meditation is defined as a state of relaxation and heightened mental awareness that occurs when the mind is calm and focused. Meditation happens when the mind is fully absorbed in the present moment, and not thinking of the past or future. There are many meditation techniques to keep the mind quiet, calm, and, peaceful.

Acceptance

Art Brownstein, M.D., writes, "No matter where in your body you experience pain, it is important not to fight with it, hate it, or be angry at it. Learn to accept, which is the first step in the healing process." Don't accept it as a permanent condition and don't run away from it. Pain creates fear which agitates the mind resulting in stress. Fear causes back muscles to tense up, which causes more pain, which cause more fear. The cycle perpetuates itself.

The pain-fear cycle can be broken in two ways. One way is to target the fear at the mental level with stress management techniques that relax the mind such as relaxation, breathing, meditation, and visualization. The muscles will relax. The second way is to stretch your muscles and practice breathing and relaxation techniques. Acceptance produces improved treatment outcomes.

Hypnosis and Imagery

Both hypnosis and imagery are states of highly focused attention in which altered states of awareness, sensation, and perception can occur. Hypnosis can reduce pain by attention control and disassociation, and may or may not include imagery or visualization. The process of hypnosis implies an effort to achieve a state of highly focused attention allowing a patient to be susceptible to suggestion. Suggestion is a very powerful tool, perhaps accounting for the placebo effect. Scientific evidence shows that highly hypnotized subjects can reduce pain significantly more than non-hypnotized subjects. Clinicians often use the term imagery because of patient bias regarding hypnosis.

Many studies have proven that imagery and hypnosis can

reduce many types of pain. Some researchers believe that hypnosis changes the pain experience by shifting attention away from bodily sensations. In a meta analysis of studies on the efficiencies of cognitive behavioral methods for pain control reported that imagery was the most powerful tool which significantly relieved various types of pain. Few controlled studies have been done on hypnotherapy for pain relief. Conditions responding to hypnosis include burn pain, migraines, and phantom limb pain. With chronic pain, hypnosis, imagery, meditation, and relaxation all have been proven effective. No studies have shown one technique to be better than another.

Group Therapy

Pain is a private experience that has important social consequences, writes Robert Gatchel. Knowing that someone is experiencing pain often affects how that person is treated. The social response affects the way pain sufferers cope with their pain.

Studies have found those who receive support and encouragement from others often have less severe pain. Psychologists have found group therapy very effective in helping patients learning to cope with chronic pain. The advantages of group therapy include:

1. Patients learn they are not alone in experiencing behavioral and psychological problems.

2. Patients better understand their pain and the role of thoughts and feelings and their influence on pain.

3. Group therapy teaches patients coping skills to deal with their pain and has become one of the major forms of treatment for chronic pain. Controlled studies have shown group therapy can reduce low back pain, rheumatoid arthritis pain, and osteoarthritis pain.

There are three major goals of group therapy.

1. Creating behavior change that will provide a new set of coping skills to reduce pain.

2. Patient education about their pain and disease, including medical and surgical treatment, and alternative therapies. This is effective for increasing patient knowledge but does not necessarily help pain.
3. Social support helps overcome feelings of isolation. The groups provide encouragement from others in the same situation.

There are two national self-help organizations that provide material to individuals wishing to start their own support group.

American Chronic Pain Association, Located in Rocklin, CA

National Chronic Pain Outreach, Located in Bethseda, MD

The mind is a wonderful healing tool. Your thoughts govern your mind, which governs your body. This is why positive thoughts are so important in the healing process of pain. The next two chapters will explore the world of back pain and the important role of the mind.

Chapter Four

Back Pain

Natural Remedies

Statistics may not be interesting, but they sure shed light on the morbidity of back pain. Back and neck pain are two of the most common pain symptoms resulting in doctor's visits. One study reported 31 percent of U.S. adults had experienced back or neck pain during the last 12 months. Another study involving British and Canadian adults found one third of the subjects had experienced back or neck pain in the last month, with 80 percent in the last six months. Further research has shown that 75 percent of people with back pain reported pain in other parts of the body, with 89 percent of neck pain sufferers reporting additional pain areas. Interestingly, only 25 percent of back and neck sufferers seek medical care in Canada and 37 percent in the United States. The majority of sufferers, 54 percent, used alternative medicine such as chiropractic, massage, relaxation therapy, and herbal medicine. Between 16 to 21 percent of back pain sufferers missed work, school, or other chores due to pain. Back pain can be expensive.

Low back pain is the most common type of chronic pain, affecting 59 percent of adults at some time in their life, being the fifth most common reason for primary care physician visits. British surveys found persisting back pain symptoms occurring 12 months after the first consultation to a physician by 42 to 74 percent of patients. In other words, traditional therapy does not always work.

Risk Factors for Back Pain

There are a number of risk factors that increase the chance of developing neck or back pain which include:

1. Being female
2. Increased age
3. Living alone
4. History of pain
5. Poor health
6. Nicotine use
7. Not a sports participant

Work related risk factors include:

1. Dissatisfaction with job
2. Neck pain risks
   a. Repetitious work
   b. Prolonged neck flexion
3. Low back pain risks
   a. Heavy lifting or pulling
   b. Prolonged standing
4. Work absenteeism greater than eight days.

Physical variables

1. Obesity
2. Restricted spine movement

Psychological factors

1. Depression
2. Anxiety
3. Stress
4. Poor coping skills

Often one cannot identify what is causing back pain. An MRI study of 89 men found 32 percent of men with no low back pain had an abnormal MRI, while 47 percent of men with low back pain had a normal spine. A seven-year prospective study did not link radiographic changes to subsequent development of low back pain.

Art Brownstein, M.D., wrote an excellent book entitled *Healing Back Pain Naturally*. Brownstein is an instructor of medicine at the University of Hawaii. He states that all back pain begins with problems in the muscles. When back muscles are tight, tense, weak, or out of balance, the slightest provocation can easily cause strain, injury, spasm, and intense back pain. The muscles are the greatest source of pain because they are directly connected to the nerves that transmit pain.

Brownstein claims that the overwhelming majority of back problems are created or made worse by stress created in the mind. If a person is under tension for a period of time, the muscles contract and become more and more tight, stiff, and painful. In other words, the back muscles automatically tighten up under stress. In the absence of an injury, with tense muscles in the spine, the back is just an accident waiting to happen, writes Brownstein. Even if the doctor said the back problem is the result of degenerating disc disease, bone spur, spinal arthritis, pinched nerve, or scoliosis or some other condition, Dr. Brownstein emphasizes that all of these conditions began with problems in the muscles of the back. Once the health of back muscles is restored, all the above conditions will be reversed, and the patient will be free of pain. By becoming aware of the importance of the mind and back muscle pain, Brownstein claims that his protocol can heal the pain and strengthen the back. No longer does one have to be incapacitated or have debilitating pain.

There are literally thousands of muscles in the back that move and support the spine. It is the back muscles that determine the health of the spine. Keeping back muscles strong, flexible, and properly balanced is the key to healing back pain. When the health of the back is in jeopardy, pain is the first warning. The function of back muscles is to protect the delicate spinal column and to align the vertebrae of the spinal column. Imbalance occurs when one of the back muscles is in pain. The muscle may be too weak, too strong, or too tense. When there is a threat to the spinal cord, the sensitive spinal muscles go into spasm and lock themselves into a tight grip. Back muscle spasm is 10 to 20 times more painful than any other muscle spasm. The back muscles are connected to about every other muscle group in the body. When the spine is unhealthy, the whole body suffers. Brownstein emphasizes that no matter how many operations one has had on the back, the muscles can be trained to do yoga, weight lifting, swimming, jogging, hiking with a backpack, gardening, and much more.

The mind generates 600 to 800 thoughts a minute. Each thought generates electrical impulses that reach the muscles in the back. Stress causes tension in the mind, which translates to tension in the back muscles. Stress also increases the number of negative thoughts. Thought transforms electrical nerve muscles to all parts of the body. Repeated negative thought stimuli cause the muscles to become tight, tense, and painful. This is how a lie detector works. Muscle tension increases when people lie, caused by increased mental effort to cover up the lie, which in turn is caused by fear and anxiety of being discovered. When pain is present, there is always hope and potential for healing, because pain means life, writes Brownstein.

If one blocks natural pain messages, one cannot hear the language of the body. Taking artificial chemicals such as drugs suppress the body's natural message of pain and can be dangerous and harmful. Endorphins and encephalins are powerful biochemicals of the nervous system that the body uses to regulate pain. They are more powerful than heroin and morphine. Exercise, laughter, and relaxation all stimulate the production of these natural pain killers. Pain forces one to change the way one thinks, feels, and acts.

Pain is as much in the mind as it is in the body, with pain receptors in the body sending a signal to the brain. The majority of back pain receptors are located in the muscles, and the exaggerated back pain sends an alarm that the spine is in trouble. Most people believe the pain is coming from a ruptured disc, pinched nerve, or other problem. It is not. It comes from the muscles. Brownstein claims the back condition will never improve until one learns to accept pain is coming from the back muscle and then learns to work with pain through stretching, strengthening, relaxing the muscles, and managing stress.

No matter where in the body you experience pain, it is important to not fight it or be angry with it. Learn to accept it, states Brownstein, as it is the first step in the healing process. Fear of pain causes stress, which causes muscles to tense up, resulting in more pain. The pain fear cycle can be broken in two ways. The first method is to break the fear cycle with the mind, through stress management that relaxes the mind, accomplished with relaxation techniques, breathing, meditation, and visualization. The second way is to stretch the muscles.

Chronic pain almost always has emotional roots. Emotions generate powerful chemistry in the body, and if the emotions are repressed, one is completely unaware of their existence. Painful and traumatic emotions get repressed at an early age and become stored in the body resulting in tension and stress and eventually pain later in life. Chronic pain is a conditioned response to deep-seated feelings of guilt or self blame. When ones feels guilty, there is an unconscious need for punishment, and this always brings pain. Dr. Brownstein believes it is much healthier to share one's emotional pain, so it can be released and be healed. Concealing pain ultimately creates more pain, and sharing emotional pain is physically healing.

Dr. Brownstein writes in his book about effective techniques to heal back pain, as he had developed chronic back pain while in medical school that almost drove him to suicide. His seven year journey to heal himself involved quitting pain drugs, doctors, and surgery. He took charge of his healing process and completely recovered by the techniques that follow. Much of this section is based on his book.

Natural Therapy for Back Pain

Stretching

All muscles affect the back in some way. Stretching is a powerful way to directly relieve pain from back muscles. Stretching releases stored up tension; it releases knots, tightness, spasm, and pain. A flexible body is more resistant to injury. Stretching is highly effective for chronic degenerative conditions of the spine resulting from injuries or trauma. The blood supply and oxygen delivery is enhanced with stretching. If pain occurs at any time while stretching, one should ease back until the pain goes away. For acute back problems, one should avoid bending forward. If pain is felt when stretching, the muscle has been stretched too far. If the pain decreases, the stretching is beneficial. Try to stretch in the morning. Dr. Brownstein's book, *Healing Back Pain Naturally*, has many stretching exercises, a must read for back pain sufferers.

Yoga is an excellent modality for stretching derived from ancient Eastern disciplines. Yoga places a great importance on a healthy spine, and classes are available in most cities. If you suffer back pain, begin with a "gentle" yoga class.

Strengthening

By strengthening the back, one can overcome fear and build confidence in your back writes Dr. Brownstein. He cautions that all injuries should be healed before starting an exercise program. Rest is important following an injury and this should be followed by stretching which delivers more oxygen and removes waste products from the injured muscle, disc, or joint. Stretching should be done for two months or longer following a back injury. Before strengthening activity, stretch the muscles that involve contracting muscles which exert a large pulling force on joints and the opposing muscles. Listen to your body at all times. Focus on strengthening the spine only after achieving a full range of motion. Don't ignore or push through pain. The following exercises will strengthen back muscles:

1. Walking
2. Swimming
3. Jogging
4. Cycling
5. Weight lifting
6. Calisthenics
7. Aerobics
8. Favorite sport such as golf, tennis, and skiing

Stress Management

Most back pain occurs just preceding, during, or shortly after a major period of stress, writes Dr. Brownstein. To heal the back, one needs to relax and manage stress. Stress causes the muscles to automatically tense. Long term stress can cause muscle tension that misaligns the back. Deep relaxation rids the body of stress, anxiety, and tension. Relaxed muscles allow blood vessels in muscles to dilate and provide more oxygen, thereby reducing inflammation and swelling. Relaxation techniques are found in chapter three of this book.

Breathing

Improved breathing provides increased oxygenation of the blood. When a person is anxious or under stress, the breathing is disturbed. Yoga emphasizes breathing.

Visualization

The brain converts images, real or imagined, into electrical impulses before transmitting them to the body in the nervous system. The body can't distinguish between real or imagined. One can image to heal the back. Visualization is described in the "Mind as Healer" chapter.

Meditation

Meditation promotes healing by calming and centering the mind. This promotes mental tranquility, relaxes the nervous system, and reduces muscle tension. The mind is quiet, calm, peaceful, and focused during meditation, and fully absorbed in the present moment.

Diet for a Healthy Back

Excess weight can affect the spine. A large belly presses on the back muscles and discs, causing tension, misalignment, and pain. Heavy people find it difficult to move around, resulting in less movement in the joints and muscles, increasing the risk for back strain. Eating becomes one of the only enjoyable activities of life, possibly elevating one's mood, and resulting in more weight gain. One should avoid fats (keep fats to 10 to 20 percent of the diet), avoid fast foods because they are usually of high fat and low fiber content, and avoid going for long periods of time without food.

If suffering from back pain, one should eliminate stimulants such as coffee, tea, and colas. Stimulants can be harmful to the back because they affect the central nervous system, which causes the back muscles to tighten. Be sure to get enough sleep, 7.5 to 8 hours, perhaps with an afternoon nap of thirty minutes. If rested, there is no need for caffeine.

Fiber is extremely helpful for people with back problems, because it absorbs toxins, reduces intestinal gas, decreases intestinal transit, and keeps bowels functioning.

Adequate fluid intake will aid the process of eliminating toxins of both the kidney and bowels. Improving bowel function can alleviate back problems.

Studies have found cultures who consume the highest amount of vegetables in their diet have the lowest rate of back problems. Vegetables contain a multitude of beneficial nutrients required for healthy back muscles and bone. One should also eat at least two servings of fruit daily for back health. A diet rich in whole grains, beans, and legumes will provide protein to nourish back muscles. Beans and legumes contain little fat or cholesterol and provide more health nutrients than animal products.

Natural Supplements for the Back

There are many supplements (see dosage in nutrition chapter) that will aid in the healing of back problems that include:

1. **Valerian root** is an excellent tranquilizer and muscle relaxant. Take before bedtime.

2. **Comfrey root** stimulates the healing process of muscles and tendons, ligaments, bone, and disc.

3. **Chamomile** acts as a tranquilizer and a mild muscle relaxant, best taken at night.

4. **Crampbark** is a muscle relaxant helpful for muscle spasm.

5. **Melatonin** normalizes circadian rhythms and helps regulate sleep.
6. **Willow bark** is both anti-inflammatory and a pain reliever.
7. **Passion flower** is a mild tranquilizer, muscle relaxant, and pain reliever.
8. **Bromelain** can help reduce inflammation and swelling in the back, especially around the discs. It has been routinely injected directly into the discs to relieve pain symptoms.
9. **Arnica** is used in homeopathy for inflammation and pain.
10. **St. John's Wort** aids in managing chronic pain and depression.
11. **Vitamin C** aids in repairing damaged muscles, tendons, bones, and ligaments.
12. **Boron** helps build strong bones.
13. **Vitamin B complex** helps build strong bones and muscles in the back.
14. **Vitamin E** helps repair damaged muscles in the back.
15. **Magnesium** builds strong bones and helps back muscles to contract and relax.
16. **Selenium** helps build strong bones and muscles in the back.
17. **Tiger balm** improves blood flow and is effective for relieving back pain. It is very effective when applied at night.

It is always wise to consult with a physician, naturopath, or herbologist when taking herbs to be sure there are no interactions with other drugs.

Work

Studies have shown conclusively the most important thing one can do if suffering from chronic back pain is to return to work as soon as possible. This helps keep the mind off problems, provides self-esteem, and allows social interaction. Ease back into work

Humor

When one laughs and is enjoying oneself, the mind is completely at rest. Endorphins and encephalins are released into the blood stream to relieve pain and promote healing. Create a sense of humor and don't be so serious, writes Dr. Brownstein.

Emotions, Spirituality, and Healing

Emotions and attitude play a very vital role in health and disease. Many studies have found the power of prayer to be effective in the healing process. The following are some suggested tips to develop a good mind set regarding back pain that Dr. Brownstein has found to be very effective:

1. Avoid blaming yourself for your back pain.
2. Don't live in fear or be afraid of pain.
3. Honor your pain as a teacher and friend.
4. Share your pain by talking about it.
5. Learn to love your back.
6. Learn to love yourself.
7. Develop healthy and loving relationships.
8. Develop harmony in your life.
9. Acknowledge a Higher Power in your life.
10. Give gratitude to the natural abundance in your life.

Specific Back Pain Disorders

Muscle Spasm
Muscle spasm is the most common cause of back injury. For instant relief, put an ice pack on the back with a towel. Gentle stretching may help with sore muscles as it loosens them up.

Disc Problems
Discs are cushions of cartilage that separate the vertebrae. A disc can slip or rupture and the contents may press against a nerve root where it exits the spinal cord. Eight out of ten people recover from disc problems within six weeks. Bed rest is recommended for two days following the initial attack plus over-the-counter analgesics. Only 1 to 3 percent of chronic low back pain is the result of disc disorders. After the initial pain begins to subside, one should begin moving. Exercise is needed to increase the circulation to the disc and to strengthen abdominal muscles. One exercise involves lying on the back with knees bent. For instant relief, apply ice packs two or three times a day. Try over-the-counter analgesics such as extra strength Tylenol or anti-inflammation medicine such as aspirin or ibuprofen.

Low Back Pain
When one is active, gravity puts more pressure on the lower spine than the upper spine. Most low back pain, according to some experts, is caused by arthritis resulting from an accumulation of wear and tear. Dr. Brownstein would disagree and say that most lower back pain results from tense muscles, not arthritis or disc disorders. After the age of 30, people start losing water from their discs and the discs begin to wear away. The vast majority of low back pain is of 'unspecified musculoskeletal' origin attributed to muscle tension.

Evidence suggests that the muscle tension causing chronic back pain results from stress or repressed emotions. Unlocking these repressed emotions often cures chronic back pain. Low back pain incidence rises with age continuing to the age of 50 to 60, with more men than women suffering from it. Back pain is the most common sickness in men and women less than 64 years old. It is also one of the costliest health conditions, accounting for 25 percent of all disability compensation in the workplace.

Only 10 to 15 percent of patients with low back pain have shown a clear cut cause for the pain. Radiological findings in the lumbar spine are poor predictors of low back pain. Fewer than 10 percent of low back pain episodes result in consultations with a family doctor. About half of simple back pain patients improve within a week, and 90 percent within a month.

For instant relief of low back pain, one should use a heating pad. Also try laying flat on the floor with knees bent and feet elevated on a chair.

Stenosis

After the age of 50, the spine can develop bone spurs because of wear and tear. The membranes may become swollen, or ruptured discs may narrow the space through which the spinal cord runs. The narrowing of the space is called stenosis. Many people with stenosis report that leaning forward and pushing a shopping cart can help relieve the pain. Doctors often prescribe strong pain killers and will sometimes inject an anesthetic into the spine. About 30 to 35 percent of stenosis patients can be helped with exercise. Surgery may be an option, which relieves pain 80 percent of the time.

Sacroiliac Pain

Up to one-third of chronic low-back pain can be linked to pelvic instability. The sacroiliac joints, also known as SI joints, are located on both sides of the pelvis and are connected to the lower portion of the spine. A healthy SI joint does not flex, and is referred to as 'gliding joint,' meaning the ligaments holding it together can shift. Certain circumstances can cause excess movement in the SI joint such as a pregnancy. For women beyond child bearing age and for men too, SI joint pain is slightly different, usually affecting one side of the pelvis leading to chronic, nagging pain of the lower back. The pain often worsens when bending over from a standing position. Sitting is another risk factor. If the pain improves when lying down, this suggests SI joints may be involved.

Jo Ann Staugaard-Jones, MA wrote an excellent article about

SI pain in the *Bottom/Line Health* magazine (November 2015). She is a former professor of kinesiology and an advanced Pilates and Haga yoga instructor. She writes that in addition to exercises, most doctors recommend the following remedies to relieve SI pain.

1. *Ice* is used to reduce inflammation which provides a brief numbing effect that temporarily reduces pain. One should ice the affected area for 15 minutes, three times a week, and alternate ice packs with a heating pad.

2. *Massage* often helps SI pain but may aggravate the pain in some patients.

3. An *SI belt* is designed to relieve overtaxed ligaments by decreasing motion around the pelvis. Some research has found the belt helps, and another study found it did not help.

4. If natural therapies do not work, one may need pain medication such as ibuprofen or topical *arnica gel*.

5. *Exercise* can relieve SI pain by balancing the strength of the muscle and tendons surrounding the joints by providing stability. One should try the following in a 10 to 15 minute routine three times a week, with relief arriving usually between three to six weeks.

    A. *Squats:* Begin by holding a five pound weight overhead, working up to ten pounds. Stand in front of a mirror with a chair behind you to assist. The weight or bar held overhead will keep the body in correct alignment. Engage your abdominal and back muscles as you bend your knees, lowering yourself toward a sitting position. Allow your hips to fall toward the chair until your buttocks lightly touch the chair. Try to position your upper thighs to be parallel to the floor. Hold the squat for 10 to 20 seconds and slowly return to standing position. Repeat three to five times.

    B. *Hand/Knee Balance:* Get down on all fours in a 'table top' position with your back as level and flat as possible. Begin by stretching your right leg back and lifting it to hip height. Then slowly lift your left arm forward in line with your ear. Keep your pelvis stable and centered by keeping your core muscles tight. Hold the position for ten seconds. Return to the tabletop position and repeat on the other side. Alternate sides for one minute.

C. *SI Stretch*: Lie on your back on an exercise mat or carpeted floor with your legs straight and arms outstretched to your sides. Bend your right knee toward your chest and then let it fall across your body to the left, letting your hips roll with it. Keep both shoulders on the floor and breath in and out for one minute before repeating on the other side.

D. Join a yoga class as some of these exercises are included in gentle yoga.

Sciatica

The sciatic nerve is the largest thickest nerve in the body. This large nerve is formed by the joining of lumbar (L4, L5) and sacrum (S 1, S 2, S 3) spinal nerve roots, which run to the lower back to the heel.

Pain in the sciatic nerve is described as sharp, piercing, hot, pins and needles, and electrical. Often it begins in the lower back and travels down the buttocks, along the side and back of leg, around the knee, and to the ankle, and then to the toes. About 90 percent of sciatica problems resolve themselves.

Sciatica is usually caused by a back disc problem, a spinal disorder that causes compression of the nerve. Some believe it is caused by a spasm of the piriformis muscle located deep inside the buttocks, but this is considered rare. The six most commons causes include:

1. Bulging or herniated disc
2. Lumbar spinal stenosis
3. Spondylolisthesis is where a vertebrae slips forward onto a bone below.

Back Pain

4. Trauma
5. Piriformis syndrome
6. Spinal tumor

Dr. Letha Hadady, D.Ac., in her book *Naturally Pain Free*, writes about natural and preventive techniques and treatment for sciatica that include:

1. Stay hydrated, especially with Gatorade which is made of 94 percent water, plus 6 percent fructose, corn syrup, citric acid, food starch, potassium sulfate, and sodium citrate.
2. A lemon foot soak will reduce inflammation.
3. Correct posture is important. One should sleep on a firm mattress.
4. Place a magnet belt over the pain area, as magnets enhance blood circulation and relieve muscle tension.
5. Eat a cleansing diet because sciatica is compounded by constipation. Ayurvedic medicine suggests a light diet of fruits, vegetables, and complex carbohydrates. Bananas and apples are good, as is turmeric which is both anti-inflammatory and antibiotic.

Alternative therapies for sciatica as mentioned in Burton Goldberg's book entitled *Alternative Medicine: The Definitive Guide* include:

1. A diet high in vitamin B1 (thiamine) and magnesium which are natural muscle relaxants that include dark leafy green vegetables, yellow vegetables, whole grains, seeds, and nuts.
2. Avoid caffeinated beverages, chocolate, and refined sugar.
3. Take supplements of magnesium, thiamine, vitamin B complex, possibly vitamin B12 injections, vitamin E, calcium, and manganese sulfate.

4. Acupressure can relieve sciatica. Lie down on your back with legs bent and feet flat on the floor. Place hands under the buttocks, palms down beside the base of spine. Close your eyes and take long deep breaths and rock your knees from side to side for two minutes to press acupressure points in the buttocks. Reposition your hands for comfort to enable different parts of the buttocks muscles to be pressed.

5. Aromatherapy is effective by applying a cold press and a light massage with chamomile or lavender.

6. Ayurveda medicine uses 200 mg of triphala guggulu, generally taken with warm water twice a day after lunch and dinner.

7. Herbs are also effective. Mix in equal parts of willow bark and St. John's Wort tincture and take one-half teaspoon three times a day. A massage with St. John's wort oil will also help alleviate pain.

8. Homeopathy remedies include colocynth, viscum album, lachesis, rhus tox, and aconite, all which may help.

9. Hydrotherapy at body temperature has a profound calming effect.

10. TENS (transcutaneous electrical nerve stimulation) treatment is effective for relief of sciatica.

One herbal combination that has been effective for sciatica is *Mobility 2*, which contains red peony, persica, tang kuei, and ligusticum, all which invigorates blood circulation. It contains a total of 17 herbs.

Controlled studies regarding sciatica and chiropractic manipulation found chiropractic therapy to be effective for pain relief.

Other Natural Therapies for Back Pain

Braces, Chairs, and Lifting

Braces and back supports are used to support oneself through the critical stages of almost any critical back problem.

Chairs should have an armrest and lumbar support. A recliner is the best type of chair.

To lift heavy objects, squat down and keep the back straight. Hold the object close to the body and use the strong leg muscles to do the lifting.

Hot and Cold Packs

Hot and cold packs can be soothing to chronically sore backs. Heat will dilate the blood vessels and improve the oxygen supply to the back to help reduce muscle spasm. Heat alters the sensation of pain, and cold reduces inflammation and can numb deep pain.

Physical Therapy

Active physical therapy with behavioral intervention is the most effective method of achieving long term pain relief in order to regain the ability to resume normal activity.

Rehabilitation

Dawn Marcus, M.D., in her book *Chronic Pain: A Primary Guide to Practical Management* states that an intensive rehabilitation program that combines active exercise with psychology therapy including coping skills, distraction techniques, and relaxation along with education are the most effective methods for improving function and reducing pain for disabled patients with chronic back pain. About half of disabled patients are able to work. However, the outcome is worse for those who receive compensation for back pain.

Chiropractic

Chiropractic is a profession dedicated to relieving back pain. Many people who have not been helped by traditional medicine often find back pain relief from chiropractors. Chiropractors will align the spine and vertebrae to give pain relief. Many studies have confirmed the efficacy of chiropractic spinal manipulation for back pain. A visit to the chiropractor is a must for back pain.

Most chronic back pain is caused by stress and repressed emotions. This has been verified by Dr. John Sarno, a professor of medicine at New York University Medical School. The next chapter will summarize three of his books regarding back pain and the mind.

Chapter Five

The Illusion of Back Pain

An Emotional Dis-ease

I believe it was sometime in 1998 when I was watching the television news magazine program *20/20*. John Stossel was narrating this particular segment regarding back pain. He began the report by relating an episode that happened on the *Rosie O'Donnell Show* months before. A show employee had severe back pain and became so incapacitated that she could only move about with an automated wheelchair. She had tried most of the traditional and alternative therapies without success. As the story goes, Rosie invited her employee onto her program to ask the national audience for their ideas on how to eliminate her excruciating chronic pain. The letters began to pour in, and one therapy rose to the top for being successful in eliminating back pain. It involved the treatment of John Sarno, M.D., a New York University physician. John Stossel devoted the remainder of the segment to the therapy program of Dr. Sarno. In fact, the producers asked Dr. Sarno if they could randomly select 20 files from his office and talk to the patients. Dr. Sarno consented, and all 20 patients said they had been cured from their chronic pain. This chapter is based on the work of John Sarno, M.D., as referenced in his three books demonstrating the principles of mind/body medicine.

The views expressed in this chapter are my own. My

discussion of the materials relating to Dr. Sarno has not been approved, sponsored, or endorsed by Dr. Sarno. Dr. Sarno's work is in depth and very subtle, and I recommend that you read his books to understand his ideas and views, and not rely on this work as a substitute or summary.

Dr. Sarno was director of patient services at the Institute of Rehabilitation Medicine at New York University Medical Center. He is now retired. His story began in the 1970s, where as a physician of rehabilitation medicine, he found it very difficult to successfully treat back pain. Between 80 to 90 percent of Americans experience pain in the back, neck, and shoulders sometime during their lifetimes. Medical science had been unable to solve this 20th century problem. Sarno found that 88 percent of back pain patients had a history of tension, migraine headaches, heartburn, stomach ulcers, colitis, spastic colon, allergies, and other common disorders, all of which are related to tension. Dr. Sarno then realized that back pain was possibly a stress problem, not a structural abnormality related to vertebrae, disks, or pinched nerves. It was a muscle condition that was probably related to tension. Sarno then put his theory to work and began to help many back pain patients. He began to predict those patients who would be helped and those who would not. It was apparent that nervous tension initiated back pain, but he was unclear about the nature of the painful process, only that muscle spasm was one of the ingredients.

Dr. Sarno then discovered that tension affected the circulation of blood to the involved area. When muscles and their associated nerves were deprived of their normal supply of oxygen, the result was pain in the back and/or limbs. He concluded that a reduction of oxygen to the muscles and nerves appears to be the direct cause of muscle and nerve pain. His hypothesis was confirmed by German scientists whose electron microscope studies of back muscle cells suggested oxygen deprivation.

Back pain has reached epidemic proportions in the Western world. It has become one of the most common disorders for which people seek medical help. Costing billions of dollars each year in medical and chiropractic costs, it is the single largest cause of worker absenteeism in the United States, Sweden, Great Britain, and Canada. Medicine has been unable to recognize the nature of the disease and unable to recognize the nature of the disease and unable to make an accurate diagnosis. For these reasons, Dr. Sarno was determined to help these suffering people.

Sarno found that, contrary to popular belief, injuries or disease of the spine are rarely responsible for pain in the neck, shoulders, or back. Because the idea that pain is due to a variety of structural abnormalities of the spine is so deeply ingrained in the medical mind set, alternative diagnoses are seldom considered. The majority of physicians do not consider that emotions play a role in causing physical disorders, but they acknowledge that emotions might aggravate a physically caused disease. Dr. Sarno disagrees with his colleagues and believes that about 90 percent of back pain is caused by emotions and tension. Because emotions and tension can lead to a physical process involving muscles and nerves of the neck, shoulder, and back, he termed this condition the tension myositis syndrome – TMS. In other words back pain is a form of TMS caused by stress, emotions, and tensions. The physical cause of back pain is an illusion.

Tension can cause constriction of the blood vessels feeding the muscles and nerves, which deprives the tissues of oxygen, resulting in nerve pain and muscle spasms. This pain can recur with increasing frequency over many years, and it finally becomes chronic for some people. As a result, TMS (back pain) patients become more anxious, increasing the internal tension that perpetuates the pain-producing process. Fear accompanies this painful syndrome: fear of physical degeneration, fear of further injury to the back, fear of disability, and fear of pain itself. Fear creates a vicious cycle. Dr. Sarno does not consider TMS a disease, because it rarely leads to significant damage to the involved nerves and muscles.

Back Conditions

Physicians and chiropractors have diagnosed a number of physical conditions that cause back pain. However, Dr. Sarno has found very few of these physical conditions to be the cause of back pain, since he has cured pain in all the following conditions with simple mind/body therapy. He claims that once a person has experienced neck, shoulder, or back pain, it will come back, regardless of type or length of treatment, but not always in the same place. Only his TMS (back pain) therapy, which treats the cause, can eliminate the pain forever.

Herniated Discs: The disks at the lower end of the spine (lumbar region) are subject to a lot of stress. Each acts as a shock absorber between two vertebrae and can wear out over time. When this occurs, the fluid within the cavity may bulge at a weak point and actually break through. At this point, it is called a herniated or ruptured disk. Usually it is blamed for leg pain called sciatica, based on case history and x-rays. However, a disk in advanced stages of degeneration cannot herniate. Of great importance, claims Dr. Sarno, is that a proven herniated disk does not cause pain in the majority of cases. He has treated many patients who have lumbar herniated disks, documented by positive mylograms and CT scans. His mind/body treatment could not have been successful if the pain had been due to disk herniation.

Dr. Sarno has successfully treated patients in which herniation was found to be compressing a spinal nerve. Patients experienced the same pain after the disk material was removed surgically. These patients had TMS and were cured of their pain by Sarno's mind/body TMS treatment. He believes that back pain patients should first be treated for TMS. If improvement occurs, the TMS diagnosis has been validated.

Often patients are told a herniated disk puts pressure on the sciatic nerve, resulting in pain. Dr. Sarno says this is an anatomical impossibility. If the herniated disk material is pressing on one of the spinal nerves that sends a branch to the sciatic nerve, the nerve could not function because of the persistent compression. It is oxygen deprivation, not nerve compression, that causes the symptoms, explaining why sciatica patients have pain in so many different parts of the leg. A structural abnormality like a herniated disk could not produce the clinical picture.

Neurosurgeon H. L. Rosomoft claims that lumbar herniations are responsible for back and leg pain in fewer than 3 percent of cases. One study reported in the *New England Journal of Medicine* concluded, "The discovery by MRI of bulges or protrusion in people with low back pain may frequently be coincidental." In 1956, Donald McRae published a paper claiming that anyone over 30 years of age may have a herniated disk without symptoms.

In 1987, Dr. Sarno studied 96 of his patients who had a herniated disk as documented by a CT scan. They had undergone the mind/body TMS treatment between 1983 and 1986. Of the 96 patients, 88 percent were cured of back pain, 10 percent improved, and 2 percent had no change. Sarno's scientific paper was rejected by seven medical journals. Does that tell you something about the bias of medical journals?

> *Pinched Nerve:* Frequently health care practitioners believe neck, shoulder, and arm pain is caused by a pinched nerve. Physicians assume that one of the spinal nerves emerging from the neck is compressed by a bone spur from one of the cervical vertebrae. Bone spurs are very common and most people who have them do not complain of pain. Young adults have similar conditions, but without pain. Chiropractors frequently believe vertebrae are out of alignment, causing the nerves to be pinched.

Dr. Sarno disagrees that this is the cause of neck, shoulder, and arm pain. He believes TMS is the cause and has successfully treated a high percentage of these pain sufferers. Often the patients experience numbness, tingling, and pain in the shoulders, neck, and arm; these are but symptoms of oxygen deprivation.

> *Other Structural Anomalies:* Arthritis in the joints of the spine is a common occurrence in the normal aging process. Frequently it is claimed to be the cause of neck and back pain. Dr. Sarno says no, as he has successfully treated many TMS patients with spinal arthritis.

Congenital anomalies, transitional vertebrae, spina bifida, and spondylitis are seen easily on X-ray. According to Dr. Sarno, none of these conditions is responsible for pain in his patients. An article by C.A. Splithoft in the *Journal of the American Medical Association* (1953) concluded that patients without backaches demonstrated structural aberrations just as frequently as patients with back pain. A later Israeli study came up with a similar conclusion. Dr. Sarno asserts that neither scoliosis nor spinal curvatures cause pain in any of his patients. He has also treated successfully with TMS therapy a number of patients who had a serious misalignment of the lower spine.

Frequently back pain patients are prescribed anti-inflammatory medication for pain relief, with physicians believing back pain is associated with inflammation. Inflammation is a reaction to most injuries and disease, but is not the cause of most back pain. There is no inflammation with ordinary neck, shoulder, or back pain — neither X-rays nor blood tests show it. In summary, most diagnoses regarding the cause of neck, shoulder, and back pain are wrong. This is quite alarming, considering the risks of surgery and medication that accompany this misdiagnosis. Billions of dollars are unnecessarily spent each year trying to eliminate a pain problem that can be cured by a simple mind/body technique!

The Cause of Back Pain

Dr. Sarno believes neck, shoulder, and back pain are related to a person's feelings, personality, and hardships of life. Back pain is a reflection of temperament. As lives become more complex, people undergo more stress, and this is why the pain is so common.

He has observed a distinct personality in his back pain (TMS) patients. Most have a type "A" personality; they are extremely compulsive about their work and responsibility, leaving little time for play and relaxation. TMS patients are conscientious people who are responsible and hard working, with a great inner drive.

Underlying back pain in these patients, claims Dr. Sarno, is repressed anger and feelings of guilt. This often leads to tension that causes back pain. Putting things out of one's mind does not get rid of them, but simply banishes them to the unconscious. Tension results from the battle going on in the subconscious mind, the conflict over doing something about the problem or ignoring it. The process of back pain then becomes self-generating, creating a vicious cycle as the pain itself develops anxiety, thereby causing more pain.

Often the doctor is not sure what causes the pain, thus creating more anxiety with a confused diagnosis. Patients are often told not to exercise, creating a fear and apprehension toward exercise, which leads to additional anxiety. Psychological factors caused by back pain may include a feeling of inadequacy: a mother cannot lift her child; a sufferer cannot sit through a movie; a father cannot play ball with his son.

There is no release of this excess tension, but the energies of tension need to be expressed in some manner. Emotion is the most logical way to vent this energy, because that is where it originated. Unpleasant feelings, the fear of conflict, and not wanting to hurt someone are some reasons why people tend to hold in these emotions. Expressions of these feelings are often not accepted by the outside world. The brain then chooses to channel this energy somewhere else, namely through the body and often the back.

The mind develops a strategy to avoid the appearance of emotional problems. The tension is channeled into the body, and a physical disorder is substituted for the repressed emotion. Because the tension from emotion is hidden, the patient feels no shame regarding the emotion. Such physical manifestations are called psychosomatic disorders, including back pain and other TMS symptoms. Other psychosomatic disorders may include a nervous stomach, gastritis, ulcer, colitis, spastic colon, hiatal hernia, tension headaches, migraine headaches, hives, eczema, hayfever, allergies, and asthma — some of the most common. Nearly 90 percent of Dr. Sarno's TMS patients have a history of one these symptoms, with 28 percent having four or more of these disorders.

A direct correlation exists between the level of tension and magnitude of pain. In other words, the more tension a person is under, the higher the pain level. Some people have higher tension levels at night, while others peak during the day.

What causes the pain? Back pain begins in the brain with a group of nerve cells that comprise the limbic system. Nearby lies the autonomic nervous system part of the brain that controls the involuntary functions of the body such as breathing, heartbeat, and digestion. It also controls blood circulation, determining what part of the body will have a normal, increased, or decreased amount of blood. Changes in blood circulation are determined by temperature, exercise, fear, stress, and anxiety. Back pain is the result of tension induced by decreased blood circulation (ischemia). Tension causes the arterioles to constrict, resulting in less blood flow which means fewer red blood cells to carry oxygen. Therefore, the tissue and muscles do not receive enough oxygen and as a result, pain manifests, be it in the lower back, shoulder, or neck. The decreased blood supply is not sufficient to damage the muscles or nerves.

As a result of constricted blood vessels, pain is first due to an accumulation of chemical waste products in the muscle. Usually these waste products are carried away and eliminated by blood, and detoxified by other parts of the body, such as the kidney. However, a sluggish circulation allows the waste products to accumulate. Reduced circulation will next cause insufficient oxygen to reach the muscles, resulting in muscle spasms. The pain can be excruciating. Decreased circulation also reduces the oxygen supply to nerves such as the sciatic nerve in the buttocks, spinal nerves in the lower back and neck, and brachial plexus nerves that innervate the arms and hands. The response to lower levels of oxygen is pain. Other ramifications may include numbness, feelings of pins and needles, and reduced strength. Oxygen deprivation to the sciatic nerve can cause pain in the buttocks and legs; oxygen deprivation to the spinal nerves can cause neck and back pain; and if the brachial plexus is affected, there may be pain in the arms and hands. Pain will be felt by any nerve deprived of oxygen.

Many of Dr. Sarno's patients believed their pain was due to an injury brought on by a physical incident, perhaps by lifting an object or being in a car accident. Following the episode, the neck or back pain started. Sarno claims these incidences are only triggers and have nothing to do with the basic cause of the pain.

In 1978, Dr. Sarno surveyed a group of 100 TMS patients to discover how their pain started. Sixty percent said their pain was not associated with a physical incident, and that it had come on gradually. The other 40 percent said there was a sudden onset — accidents (18 percent), strain (18 percent), twist (10 percent), and other (4 percent). In the 60 percent group, there was no possible correlation between a physical incident and onset of pain. Within the 40 percent group, Dr. Sarno found no relationship between how the pain began and its severity and longevity.

He concluded that physical incidents did not cause the pain, but acted as triggers. The process of TMS (tension myositis syndrome) existed in the back muscles for months or years before the pain started, but at some critical point, the pain began. In 40 percent it was associated with a physical stimulus, and in 60 percent it came out of nowhere.

For muscle sprains, tears, or strains, healing takes place in a matter of days or weeks. However, in patients who are convinced they have injured their backs, the pain will continue to exist. Dr. Sarno has discovered if patients can be made aware that the pain is caused by tension, the problem will be resolved. In other words, if the patient believes there is a physical problem, the pain will persist. Once they realize it is not the result of an injury, but a physical/emotional response to financial problems, job stress, or marital problems, the pain will leave.

About two-thirds of TMS patients will have the primary pain in the muscles of the lower back and buttocks region; 28 percent will have the primary problem in the neck muscles, shoulders, and upper back; and 8 percent will complain of the primary location in the small of the back, the lumbar region. If nerves are involved, the most common location for pain is in the legs and arms, in that order.

Because the pain is due to tension, the level of tension will vary from day to day, and the pain will also vary. If the pain were due to a structural abnormality, such as an arthritic spur, pain would be expected to be the same. TMS involves many more muscles than those that hurt spontaneously. In 100 patients with TMS, Dr. Sarno found tenderness in the neck, buttocks, and shoulder in three-fourths of the patients. He concluded that only postural muscles and associated nerves are targets for tension. Muscle tenderness from light pressure is the hallmark sign of TMS.

Repressed Emotions

The concept of repressed emotions and the unconscious are closely tied together. The reason for repression is that a person wants to avoid what is emotionally unpleasant. There is an equally strong force in the mind that is working to bring those feelings to consciousness. Frequently, back pain or TMS arises from anxiety, anger, and resentment, with the origins often occurring in childhood. About 80 percent of the United States population has a history of these pain syndromes, and Dr. Sarno has seen the incidence increase geometrically during the past four decades. He believes the role of the pain syndrome is not to express the hidden emotions, but to prevent them from becoming conscious.

The pain of TMS (back pain) is created in order to distract the attention of the sufferer from what is going on in the emotional sphere. It is intended to focus one's attention on the body instead of the mind. TMS provides a way to keep those antisocial, unkind, childish, angry, and selfish feelings from becoming conscious, claims Dr. Sarno. Defenses against repressed emotions work by diverting one's attention to something other than emotions that are being hidden in the unconscious. TMS is one such defense. Back, neck, and shoulder pain has been the preferred defense against the repressed emotion. No one suffering from these pain syndromes believes they are related to emotional factors.

Back pain occurs because people are coping very well with repressed emotion that might be otherwise interfering with their lives. Back pain exists in order to maintain repression of those emotions. According to Dr. Sarno, the TMS personality needs to be loved, admired, and respected. These people have a drive to achieve and are intensely competitive. Back pain is very rare in indigenous Africans, perhaps they are not as anxious as their American counterparts. However, back pain is just as common in Caucasians and Asians around the world as it is in the United States and Canada.

Another group of disorders has been discovered by Dr. Sarno as part of the TMS repertoire. These, thought to be soft tissue pathology, include the disorders of fibromyalgia, fibrositis, and myofascitis. They are often attributed to injury or muscle incompetence, the perfect camouflage for repressed emotions. As long as the person's attention is focused on the pain syndrome, there is no danger that the emotion will be revealed. Other TMS equivalents include digestive disorders, headaches, hypoglycemia, skin problems, allergies, and asthma, to name only a few. Each of these physical conditions serves equally to assist in repression of emotions. Physical defenses are opposed to psychological defenses and are the most common and successful defense. They are very effective because they can transfer from one disorder to another, claims Dr. Sarno. As a result, the mind simply shifts to another disorder such as headaches to digestive disorders. An interesting example of this scenario concerns ulcers as written about by Russell Baker in the *New York Time Magazine* (August 16, 1981) titled "Where Have all the Ulcers Gone?" The article suggests that physicians and lay people alike had come to realize that ulcers really meant tension. Ulcers no longer serve the purpose of hiding tension and so fewer people develop them.

Dr. Sarno believes that any organ or system in the body can be used by the mind as a defense against repressed emotions, including immune system disorders. One academic urologist believes that 90 percent of prostatitis cases are due to tension.

The overall severity of the pain syndrome is a good guide to the importance of the underlying emotional state of the patient. It may be a barometer of how much anger and anxiety the person has or how severe the trauma of early life that has contributed to the person's psychological state was. People who were abused as children have gigantic reservoirs of anxiety and anger lying within. Many sexually abused children carry great fear and rage in their minds in adulthood that they dare not acknowledge. Dr. Sarno found that 95 percent of TMS patients have mild reasons for their anxiety, and when the pain disappears, they have no adverse emotional reaction. Anything that heightens anxiety, such as fear, will increase the severity of the symptoms.

A person has three minds — conscious, unconscious, and subconscious. The conscious mind has the traits of being logical, thoughtful, controlled, independent, concerned for others, and confident and deals with morality, guilt and striving to be good. In contrast, the unconscious mind includes the traits of being irrational, emotional, willful, dependent, and fearful and exhibits feelings of rage, amorality, and low self-esteem. The subconscious mind includes the realm of perception, cognition, reason, judgment, and creativity.

The conscious mind copes well with personality-imposed pressures of daily life. It is the internal reaction to the pressures that leads to accumulated rage and the threat that the rage will erupt into the conscious. Rage in the unconscious is perceived as dangerous and threatening. As a result, there may be a dramatic overreaction in the form of pain and other physical symptoms. TMS teaches us that only feelings that the mind perceives as dangerous are repressed, inducing physical reactions. Consciously suppressed anger contributes to the reservoirs of rage in the unconscious, according to Dr. Sarno. Anger can also be generated in the unconscious as a result of internal conflict, the stress of life, or perhaps negative childhood experiences. In summary, unconscious anger, repressed anger, and suppressed anger all play a role in TMS and back pain.

The intensity of anger, up to the point of rage, determines the necessity for physical symptoms as a diversion. The threat that rage will explode into the consciousness must be of a sufficient magnitude to warrant production of TMS or one of its equivalents.

Symptoms then become players in the strategy to keep attention focused on the body so as to prevent dangerous feelings from escaping into consciousness. This avoids a confrontation with feelings that are unbearable. Because the unconscious is often illogical and irrational and is terrified by the rage, it reacts to keep the emotion repressed by employing physical symptoms. However, powerful emotions like rage continue to strive to reach consciousness.

Once patients become aware of rage or unbearable feelings, their feelings cease the struggle to become conscious. Allowing conscious awareness removes the threat of an eruption of feelings and eliminates the need for physical distraction. The pain stops! Dr. Sarno believes that rage is the principal emotion in the syndrome of back pain. However, other strong, objectionable feelings can be repressed, and may manifest as physical symptoms.

Because anger and rage are the principal players in back pain, it might be wise to explore these dangerous emotions. Back pain patients are often a type "A" personality, and traits of this personality type include anger and hostility. Hostility is overt manifestation of repressed rage or suppressed anger. Other symptoms of the type "A" personality might include anxiety, depression, or hostility, symptoms equivalent to each other.

Often the TMS patient will have low self-esteem. These patients are perfectionists and often establish standards for themselves they cannot meet. They want everyone to like them, so they need to be good. The narcissistic self reacts with anger at this imposition. TMS patients are often dependent, a trait the self views as inappropriate. Dependence becomes repressed. Because TMS patients are unconsciously dependent, this leads to unconscious rage. Often an unconscious dependency may lead to poor choices, such as a mate who will mother too much, or perhaps choosing a career that provides security but not a fulfilling challenge.

Stresses of life can generate an unconscious anger, perhaps a marriage, a divorce, pregnancy, sex difficulties, etc. Both positive and negative stress can generate unconscious anger. Accumulated anger leads to rage, and unconscious rage leads to the development of physical symptoms. So why did the pain start now? Dr. Sarno believes that when rage has reached a critical level, it threatens to erupt into consciousness, which results in back pain. There is always a therapeutic value in helping patients identify the source of rage, a fundamental principle underlying TMS.

Equivalency

Back pain, which is part of the TMS disorder, is one of a group of interchangeable physical disorders. They all serve the mind/body purpose and are equivalent to each other. We have discussed a number of equivalents — immune disorders, gastrointestinal disorders, skin problems, headaches, and infections. Most often, they will occur in tandem with TMS symptoms — 88 percent of the patients in Sarno's survey had more than one disorder. Anxiety and depression are also equivalents of TMS, serving to distract from the underlying repressed emotion. Fear is another important equivalent that may be more effective than pain itself to distract attention from repressed rage. Whatever form it takes, the mind is interested only in keeping one's attention on the body. Psychological disorders such as panic disorders and obsessive/compulsive disorders are both TMS equivalents, both reactions to anger that is either repressed or suppressed.

Immune system disorders are considered to be a TMS

equivalent. Included are allergies such as hayfever and food allergies. Frequent colds, urinary tract infections, recurrent herpes simplex, yeast infections, and prostatitis are examples of inadequate immune response to foreign invaders — TMS equivalents. The Epstein-Barr virus is affected by psychological factors. A 1994 study published in the *Journal of Consulting and Clinical Psychology* reported a decrease in Epstein-Barr titers after people were given the opportunity to write or speak about repressed feelings. Another study found that after people wrote about a stressful event, the number of their lymphocytes increased.

Chronic fatigue syndrome (CFS) is a part of the TMS disorder, consisting of fatigue, nonspecific aches and pains, and chronic infections that have been difficult to treat by medicine, leaving physicians frustrated. No lab tests or physical signs can help with the diagnosis. These people have difficulty concentrating, are depressed, and have mood disturbances. One study found that over half the people with CFS have one of the following symptoms: depression, sleep disturbance, poor concentration, worthless feelings, suicidal thoughts, and appetite and weight changes. About 25 percent suffer from anxiety.

Somewhat related to CFS is fibromyalgia, which Dr. Sarno labels as a severe form of TMS. These patients have painful muscles and psychological symptoms. Often they are anxious and depressed, have sleep problems, and lack energy. Muscle tender points are found all over the body. The pain is widespread, virtually on the entire trunk of the body, both front and back. Pain is also found in the arm and leg muscles. The symptoms suggest there is a high level of repressed emotion, especially anger, that is causing the symptoms.

Swedish scientists reported evidence of decreased oxygen levels in the muscles of people with fibromyalgia. A follow-up paper reported that by blocking the sympathetic nerves to the painful muscles, the pain would disappear. The nerve block allowed the blood supply of the muscles to return to normal. Females outnumber males ten to one with this syndrome. Dr. Sarno has successfully treated a large number of fibromyalgia patients, and their medical histories and physical examinations were consistent with severe TMS. His diagnoses were correct, since the patients recovered completely. Mild oxygen deprivation in their muscles caused the pain, supporting the hypothesis of a TMS disorder.

TMJ (temporomandibular joint syndrome) is also a part of the TMS disorder. Joint abnormalities of the jaw are the results of the symptoms rather than the cause, claims Dr. Sarno. It is much like back pain and fibromyalgia, psychogenic.

Repetitive stress injury (RSI) is another TMS disorder, and Dr. Sarno has cured many of these patients with his simple mind/body therapy. He writes, "Like the low back pain problem, misdiagnosis and mismanagement have caused repetitive stress injury to assume epidemic proportion… In 1993, it was estimated that RSI was costing corporate America $20 billion a year and was responsible for 56 percent of work related illness." Over the past several decades, carpal tunnel syndrome has become a very common disorder of RSI, largely because it was thought to be related to typing on the computer keyboard. Between 1989 and 1994, there was a 46 percent increase in disability claims from carpal tunnel syndrome. Symptoms include pain, numbness, and tingling in the wrist and hand, attributed to compression of the median nerve by a band across the wrist, the flexor retinaculum. Dr. Sarno does not agree with this etiology, but believes the disorder is better explained by a minor abnormality of TMS.

Tendons are also a target for TMS. Any tendon of the body can become the location for TMS symptoms, some more frequently than others. Dr. Sarno has successfully treated tennis elbow, foot tendinitis, shin splints, and pulled hamstrings with the TMS program of education, his mind/body therapy. He calls the MRI a mixed blessing because it is used for identifying, among other things, herniated disks, a torn meniscus in knees, or a damaged rotator cuff in the shoulder. All depend on the MRI for identification, but result in needless surgery that could be treated by TMS mind/body therapy.

Chronic pain is one of the most severe forms of TMS, claims Sarno. In 1992, Dr. John Loeser from the University of Washington said, "All the evidence suggests that for most people chronic pain is a stress-related disorder, just like ulcers. The difference with pain is that we don't know where to put the tube to look." Traditional medicine believes that chronic pain is due to psychological factors, meaning the patient was deriving secondary gain of some sort from the pain, such as avoiding responsibility. Even pain from Lyme disease is TMS, claims Dr. Sarno. Lyme disease, acquired through the bite of a tick, is a bacterial infection that manifests as neurological and arthritic symptoms.

Dr. Sarno has observed that people will develop a mind/body manifestation that is in vogue. For example, 50 years ago the stress of life may have produced ulcers and headaches. Today, the vogue disorders include back pain, repetitive stress injury, chronic fatigue syndrome, and fibromyalgia. Harold Schraeder published a study in the *Lancet* medical journal about the explosion of chronic whiplash in Norway. There were 70,000 cases — in a country of 4.2 million people — who believed they had a chronic disability because of whiplash, termed "mass hysteria" by Schraeder. Scandinavian researchers then went to investigate whiplash in Lithuania, but found that whiplash was unknown in that country, confirming the psychogenic nature of whiplash, a vogue disorder in Norway.

TMS is neither a disease nor an illness. It is a symptomatic state that is induced by the brain for a psychological purpose. The purpose of pain is to distract attention from frightening and threatening emotions and to prevent their expression, according to Columbia University psychiatrist, Stanley Coen. TMS is but one of a group of interchangeable disorders, all serving the same mind/body purpose, all equivalent to each other. Between 1973 and 1998, Dr. Sarno has seen about 10,000 patients with TMS. Most have been rendered pain-free and have assumed full physical activity. He believes that therapeutic success is more than a reasonable test of validity; it is proof of an accurate diagnosis. Fortunately for millions of sufferers, Dr. Sarno has developed a therapy program that is simple and effective. There is hope!

THERAPY FOR TMS

Just think of the countless billions of dollars that people have paid out trying to find the cause and cure of their back pain or equivalent TMS disorder. Many people have suffered in pain for years, taking medications that often have serious side effects and even death. As we have shown, the cause of these disorders is the mind trying to repress a hurtful emotion. The cause is in the mind, and the healer is also in the mind. Dr. Sarno has a track record showing that his simple mind/body therapy does work in a very effective and rapid way. As an added benefit, it costs very little money.

TMS is an emotionally induced symptom that can be removed with a drug or placebo. One of two things can happen. The symptoms will return when the drug is withdrawn or an equivalent symptom will take its place. The mind/body symptom exists to serve a purpose. If one symptom disappears, the brain will simply find a substitute symptom or disorder. This is why the treatment of symptoms does not work. To cure the disorder, one needs to treat the cause. As Dr. Sarno has shown, the cause is in the mind, a repressed emotion. The disorder is psychogenic, exacerbated by fear and anxiety. Psychogenic symptoms produce no physiologic changes in the body with TMS, as the entire process takes place in the cerebrum of the brain. The brain involves the autonomic nervous system and immune system in order to produce symptoms; the symptoms are often centered around the hypothalamus. Symptoms are not the result of disease or damage of specific body parts. They can be perceived as pain, weakness, and numbness only because the appropriate brain cells have been fired off. In other words, the symptoms are created by the brain.

The treatment of TMS (back pain and its equivalents) begins with a screening, which is followed by a consultation with Dr. Sarno. Following the consultation, patients attend two, two-hour lectures, the first on the anatomy and physiology of TMS, the second on the psychology and treatment. Following these four steps in treatment, in about 80 percent to 85 percent of patients, symptoms disappear within a matter of weeks. Those who continue to have significant pain are invited to attend weekly meetings. If the weekly meetings do not help, psychotherapy is recommended. Only about 5 percent of Dr. Sarno's patients continue to have pain, with the rate of a permanent cure between 90 percent and 95 percent. He has also discovered that many people suffering from TMS pain are helped by just reading his books.

Only after patients learn the facts about TMS will their pain go away. It is the brain that generates the physical manifestations of unaccepted emotions, in order to prevent the conscious mind from being aware of the unpleasant emotion. In his therapy, Dr. Sarno convinces the conscious mind that TMS is not serious and not worth the attention. As a result, TMS becomes useless and no longer has the ability to attract the attention of the conscious mind. The defense becomes a failure. Before the therapy can be successful, the patient has to believe in a mind/body connection. If not, the therapy will fail. Dr. Sarno will screen his patients for this belief system before accepting them in the program.

The patient then needs to acquire knowledge and act on that knowledge to change the brain behavior. The program's strategy is to provide knowledge into the nature of the disorder, followed by the patient changing his or her brain behavior. When pain sufferers become aware of the pain, they must consciously shift their attention to something psychologically negative. For example, the patient should think about a chronic family or financial problem or a recurrent source of irritation. This sends a message to the brain that the patient is no longer deceived by the brain.

The majority of Dr. Sarno's patients will have resolution of most of their symptoms in two to six weeks following the lectures. So why doesn't the pain go away immediately? Sarno believes the subconscious mind is slow and deliberate, and does not quickly accept new ideas. In contrast, the conscious mind is swift. If the patient becomes discouraged, the time for resolution may become prolonged. It also depends on how strong the repressed emotion is and how long it takes one to reject the belief that the pain is caused by a structural problem. Patients are encouraged to talk to their brains, to assert themselves, and to tell their brains they will not tolerate this state of affairs.

The most important factor, and the most difficult, is that the TMS patient must resume all physical activity. They must pursue the most vigorous activity and overcome the fear of bending, lifting, and jogging. Patients must learn to work through the fear in order to liberate themselves from the fear of physical activity. The purpose of TMS is to keep the mind from focusing on emotional things, and if the patient cannot do this, TMS symptoms will recur.

In the early years of his practice, Dr. Sarno prescribed physical therapy and medication, like Valium, to relax the muscles. He now has discontinued that protocol. Prescribing physical therapy contradicts the real cause of the disorder and emphasizes the structural explanation. The patient must remove any structural explanation for the pain, otherwise the symptoms will continue. Dr. Sarno insists that his patients cease spinal manipulation, heat, massage, exercises, and acupuncture; they all emphasize the condition is a physical disorder that can be treated by some physical means. This whole idea has to be repudiated. One should exercise for the sake of good health, but not as a remedy for the disorder.

Patients are given a list of twelve key thoughts to serve as a daily reminder. The first thing to acknowledge is that the patient understands and accepts the diagnosis — a repressed emotion. Even if a person accepts 90 percent of the diagnosis, but is concerned that possibly the herniated disk is the cause, the brain will allow the TMS to continue. Dr. Sarno believes the secret of recovering from TMS is not changing oneself, but coming to grips with the reality that one's personality can generate a great amount of anxiety and anger. The cure will occur when the patient acknowledges these unacceptable sub-conscious feelings.

CONCLUSION

Dr. Sarno's research has demonstrated that tension myositis syndrome (TMS) or backache is a remarkable example of the mind/body connection. Most physicians see illness as a disorder in the body's mechanics, and their role is discovering the defect and correcting it. Emotions are seldom considered as a cause — what cannot be studied in a laboratory is considered unscientific. Decades ago, Sigmund Freud concluded that symptoms exhibited by patients with hysteria were the result of a subconscious process of repressed painful emotions that manifested physically. He believed the symptoms were symbolic, representing a discharge of emotional tension. Freud was the first great proponent of the mind/body connection.

Many psychiatrists began to view themselves as biological psychiatrists, believing that all emotional problems were caused by chemical imbalances of the brain. Once the chemical defect was discovered, the mental disorder could be cured by a drug.

Depression and anxiety were simply derangements of brain

chemicals. Dr. Sarno disagrees with this analysis; he believes the chemical imbalance is not the cause but the result of the emotional state. He thinks these psychiatrists are practicing poor medicine by treating the symptoms and not the cause. Sadly, modern medicine has ignored the great work of Dr. Sarno. He has clinically demonstrated on thousands of patients that a physical-pathological process is the result of an emotional process, and can be halted by a mental one. Franz Alexander, the great mind/body researcher, also believes all illness is influenced in some way by the emotions. Dr. Sarno agrees, saying, "Emotions play a role in all aspects of health and illness." All medical studies are flawed if they do not consider the emotional factor, claims Sarno. Many of a person's emotional patterns are well established since childhood, before an individual becomes responsible. What they have evolved into is the result of a combination of factors — genetic, developmental, and environmental — over which a person has no control. As a result of these differences, a patient with the same psychological diagnosis may develop different TMS disorders that are mediated by the autonomic system, or by the immune system, or by psychogenic pain. Nothing in medical training has prepared the physician for this new medical paradigm.

Dr. John Sarno has discovered a whole new paradigm in health care, with clinical successes documenting the mind/body connection. Will Western medicine suppress this safe and inexpensive therapy, just because physicians do not understand it and cannot charge for it? Too many beneficial drugless therapies have followed this avenue to oblivion. Perhaps the public needs to put pressure on the medical profession to learn about Dr. Sarno's discovery. Perhaps Dr. Sarno could franchise his methodology and train non-physicians to administer this healing modality. Perhaps videotapes of lectures and consultations, along with his books, could be marketed to TMS sufferers. His discovery must not be forgotten! I tip my hat to this remarkable physician.

Chapter Six

Arthritis Pain

There May Be A Cure

The number of people who suffer from arthritis is amazing as shown by statistics from the Centers for Disease Control and Prevention. Statistics may not be exciting but I think it is wise for the reader to understand the magnitude of this painful disease.

Prevalence of Arthritis

An estimated 52.5 million adults in the United States have been told by their physician they have some form of arthritis, be it osteoarthritis, rheumatoid arthritis, gout, lupus, or fibro-myalgia. In 2012, 49.7 percent of adults over the age of 65 reported a diagnosis of arthritis. By 2030, 67 million Americans over 18 years old are projected to be diagnosed with arthritis. One in every 250 children have arthritis.

Lifetime Risk of Osteoarthritis

Nearly 50 percent of the population may develop symptomatic knee arthritis by the age of 85. Two of three obese people will develop knee arthritis, and one in four people will develop painful hip arthritis during their life.

Prevalence of Specific Types of Arthritis

In 2005, 27 million adults had osteoarthritis, the most common form of arthritis. Rheumatoid arthritis adults numbered 1.5 million in 2002. Three million adults had gout in 2002, and 6.1 million had it sometime during their life. An estimated 5 million adults had fibromyalgia in 2005.

Prevalence by Gender and Weight

One study found 26 percent of adult women had arthritis in the United States compared to 19.1 percent of men. In the study, 15.9 percent of normal or underweight adults had arthritis, compared to 22.6 percent of overweight adults and 31.2 percent of obese Americans. Another obesity study found 66 percent of overweight/obese adults had arthritis compared with 53 percent of adults without arthritis.

Physical Activity

Nearly 44 percent of adults with diagnosed arthritis reported no leisure time physical activity compared with 36 percent of adults without arthritis. One study found 44 percent of adults with knee osteoarthritis who engaged in physical activity at least three times per week were able to reduce their arthritis-related disability by 47 percent.

Disability and Hospitalization

Arthritis and other rheumatoid conditions are the major cause of disability among American adults. Approximately one in three people between the ages of 18 and 64 reported arthritis-attributed work limitation. In 2004, 3 percent of all hospitalizations were due to a primary diagnosis of arthritis. There were 78 million ambulatory visits to a physician with a primary diagnosis of arthritis. In 2003, the total cost attributed to arthritis and rheumatic conditions in the United States was $128 billion. Earning losses were $47 billion.

Mental

Arthritis is strongly associated with major depression, with the attributable risk being 18.1 percent. Nearly 7 percent of adults with arthritis report severe psychological distress.

Joint Replacement

In 2004, 454,652 total knee replacements were performed, primarily for arthritis. That same year found 232,857 hip replacements, 41,934 shoulder replacements, and 12,055 other joint replacements. I told you that statistics were not exciting but at least you now have an idea how prevalent arthritis is in the United States. The good news is that arthritis can be effectively managed without drugs according to Vijay Vad, M.D., in his book *Arthritis RX*.

Osteoarthritis

Arthritis was formerly called degenerative joint disease with the common symptoms of pain, inflammation, and limited movement of the joints. In osteoarthritis, the cartilage that covers and cushions the ends of the bone degenerate, thus allowing the bones to rub together. Pain is the primary symptom with inflammation developing later. However, one scientific source states inflammation is present in the beginning. About 2 percent of the population under 45 years of age have osteoarthritis, 30 percent between the ages of 45 and 64, and 85 percent over 65 years. In 2005, 27 million Americans had osteoarthritis. At an earlier age, more men suffer from osteoarthritis than women because they engage in more strenuous activity. However, past the age of 55 years more women suffer from it.

X-rays can diagnose osteoarthritis by showing bone change just beneath the cartilage. In advanced cases, bone spurs develop with signs of abnormal denseness, and there are pockets of fluid in the bone. Osteoarthritis begins in the articular cartilage, which is 65-80 percent water. It is a smooth glistening, bluish-white substance attached to the end of the bone. Cartilage reduces friction caused by one bone rubbing against another. During everyday life, cartilage helps protect against contact trauma on bones. When at rest, cartilage soaks up liquid called synovial fluid. This liquid is squeezed out when there is pressure. After a period of time, osteoarthritis can dry out the cartilage. As the condition progresses, the cartilage begins to soften and crack as shown by x-rays.

Symptoms of osteoarthritis include pain, stiffness, crackling, enlargement, and deformation of the affected joint.

Inflammation develops during the process. Pain begins as a minor ache and then appears only after the joint has been used. Stiffening can also occur, especially in the morning. Crepitus (joint crackling) occurs in advanced stages caused by joints rubbing together, and deformity may later develop. Osteoarthritis can affect any joint, with finger joints being a primary location.

There are two forms of osteoarthritis. The most common is the primary form, which is slow and progressive usually striking after the age of 45 years. This type mostly affects the weight-bearing joints of the knees and hips, as well as the lower back, neck, shoulders, and fingers. Primary osteoarthritis develops in two ways. One is when excessive loads are placed on normal joint tissue or when reasonable loads are applied to inferior joint tissue. About six million osteoarthritis patients have defective DNA that increases the risk. Obese people are more likely to develop osteoarthritis compared to those of normal weight. This excessive weight can become difficult to bear. Studies have shown middle-aged women can greatly reduce the risk of developing osteoarthritis simply be losing weight. Dr. Jason Theodosakis, M.D., in his book *The Arthritis Cure* states most doctors believe osteoarthritis is both inevitable and incurable. Dr. Theodosakis strongly disagrees.

Secondary osteoarthritis usually occurs before the age of 40, caused by traumatic injury, joint infection, metabolic imbalances like gout, or by joint surgery. In young people, trauma is the major cause, such as repetitive impact that occurs in sports. It is important to understand, regular exercise does not predispose a person to osteoarthritis. In fact, evidence suggests it prevents primary arthritis. Vigorous exercise actually increases the functional status of those with osteoarthritis.

Collagen is an important part of the cartilage that provides it with elasticity and the ability to absorb shock. Collagen is viewed as the 'glue' holding the cartilage matrix together. Cartilage holds the proteoglycans in place. This is a large molecule containing both protein and sugar whose purpose is to make cartilage resilient by allowing it to stretch and bounce back after movement. Proteoglycans also trap water needed for proper function. Chondrocytes are found throughout the cartilage matrix producing new collagen and proteoglycans.

In osteoarthritis, the surface of the damaged cartilage becomes ragged and pockmarked, eventually wearing completely through, allowing bones to rub against each other. As the joint lining degenerates, the joint lining called synovium often becomes inflamed. In turn, the synovium tries to resolve the situation by producing more synovial fluid that lubricates the cartilage, which then floods the joint space, causing the joint to swell resulting in more pain.

There are several theories on what causes primary osteoarthritis including:

1. A change in the cartilage matrix
2. An unchecked enzyme found in the cartilage may be out of control
3. Trauma to the subchondral bone triggers the condition
4. Perhaps a bone disease
5. An abnormal liver

Traditional Treatment for Osteoarthritis

The primary drugs for treating osteoarthritis are NSAIDs (nonsteroid anti-inflammatory drugs). Annually there are over 70 million prescriptions given to arthritis patients. This does not include the 30 billion over the counter NSAIDs sold annually. The most common NSAIDs include aspirin, celecoxib, diclofenal, etodolac, fenoprofen, ibuprofen, indomethacin, ketoprofen, ketoralac, nabumetone, and naproxen. These drugs interrupt the normal action of an enzyme called cyclooxygenase, which leads to the reduction of pain and swelling.

Studies have shown that some NSAIDs can actually damage cartilage and worsen joint function. NSAIDs can also hinder the reformation of new cartilage. Side effects of NSAIDs include gastrointestinal bleeding, impairment of cardiac function, asthma, and ulcers. Between 15 and 20 percent of patients taking NSAIDs for chronic pain have adverse gastrointestinal reactions, with nearly 100,000 Americans hospitalized annually from gastrointestinal bleeding due to NSAIDs. Approximately 16,500 deaths occur annually because of complications from NSAIDs.

The arthritis drugs Celebrex and Vioxx are even more dangerous drugs than NSAIDs because of cardiovascular complications. They target the activity of cox-2, a cyclooxygenase enzyme involved in inflammation. These two drugs can cause heart attacks, strokes, and sudden death. It is estimated that vioxx killed 60,000 people and caused at least 100,000 heart attacks before it was removed from the market in 2004. Within six months after removal, cardiovascular mortality dropped by 50,000. A 2004 study on celebrex found that 400 mg a day doubled the risk of heart attack and 800 mg increased the risk by 300 percent.

If the pain becomes unbearable, joint replacement is an option. About 25 percent of all rheumatoid arthritis patients undergo total joint replacement, with 25 percent requiring surgical repair of the joint within one year and 50 percent within seven years. Joint replacements usually last between 12 and 25 years before they cease to function and need to be replaced. The failure rate in hip replacement is significantly higher than knee replacement.

Osteoarthritis and Natural Remedies

By the age of 40, about 90 percent of individuals have x-ray evidence of osteoarthritis in their hips and knees, writes Vijay Vad, M.D., in his book *Arthritis RX*. There is no predictable correlation between x-rays, amount of pain and loss of motion. A person who shows little arthritis on x-rays may have a lot of pain. Dr. Vad has treated successfully over 5,000 patients with arthritis in their hips and knees. He has combined joint lavage with injection of hylan plus alternative therapies. A joint lavage is a non-surgical procedure that takes 15 minutes and results in a clean joint devoid of arthritis debris that provides an immediate increase in flexibility and some pain relief. Hylan is an artificial joint lubricant. The success rate of hylan injections increases from 50 percent in one year to 80 percent if joint lavage is performed prior to injection of hylan. Dr. Vad's arthritis Rx plan is a complete regimen based on exercise, diet, and supplementation. He has discovered that a diet full of refined sugar, fat, a sedentary lifestyle, and minimal exercise has led to an increase in arthritis.

Dr. Vad states one can learn to manage the pain of osteoarthritis and slow its progression with natural remedies. His Rx plan is designed to help patients live with arthritis without resorting to surgery. The plan involves minimizing risk factors that can slow its progression, which is done by exercise, diet, and supplements. Patients can reverse changes in cartilage with an emphasis on flexibility, strength, and endurance. Dr. Vad has found the people who are likely to develop osteoarthritis fall in the following categories.

1. *Heredity:* Osteoarthritis tends to run in families.
2. *Obesity:* The heavier a person is, the greater the pressure on hips and knees and other weight bearing joints. The Nurse Health Study found women who were overweight at age 18 were five times more likely to develop hip arthritis in middle age. About two thirds of adults are overweight with one third obese. A study conducted at Boston University found that obese women could decrease the risk of developing knee arthritis by just losing 11 pounds. Each pound of extra weight actually adds four pounds of pressure to knee joints.
3. *Trauma:* Severe trauma can cause cartilage damage, taking up to a year to develop osteoarthritis. There may be changes in the bone below the cartilage that don't occur as an aging process.
4. *Aging:* Experts say that aging per se isn't responsible for osteoarthritis. Cartilage does lose water content in the aging process, but it can lose water content more rapidly in an arthritic joint.
5. *Estrogen:* Following menopause, the estrogen levels in the body plummet. Estrogen replacement therapy may have a protective effect on bone in older women. Risks of estrogen therapy may include breast cancer, heart attacks, and strokes.
6. *Calcium and Vitamin D:* Calcium is essential for healthy bones, and vitamin D is necessary for calcium absorption. Diets low in calcium and vitamin D can lead to

osteoporosis. Currently, studies are trying to determine if calcium and vitamin D are linked to osteoarthritis.

7. *Occupation*: Workers who do heavy physical labor are more at risk for damaging joints that may lead to osteoarthritis. Higher risk occupations for knee arthritis include furniture movers, dock workers, and miners.

8. *Sport Injuries:* Contact sports can lead to osteoarthritis. For those who suffer meniscus tears, fractures, and ligament injuries often develop osteoarthritis of the knees. Those who play football, soccer, tennis, racket ball, and who run increase their risk of osteoarthritis.

Glucosamine and Chondroitin

Glucosamine

Glucosamine is a primary ingredient of the water-loving proteoglycan molecule, essential to make the glycosaminoglycans (Gabo) protein that binds water in the cartilage complex. Glucosamine also acts as stimulant to cells that produce chondrocytes, causing chondrocytes to produce more collagen and proteoglycans in the body. Also, it assists the body to repair damaged and eroded cartilage resulting in reduced pain and improved joint function.

Glucosamine is a nonprescription supplement that comes in four forms: sulfate, hydrochloride, hydroiodide, and n-actyl. Studies in Portugal compared glucosamine sulfate against ibuprofen known as Advil, Motrin, Nuprin, and other brand names. A double blind study was conducted on 40 arthritic patients who were given either 15 grams of glucosamine sulfate or 1.2 g of ibuprofen for eight weeks. Pain levels dropped significantly in both groups during the first two weeks. Ibuprofen had quicker pain relief than glucosamine but after two weeks ibuprofen seemed to lose its strength and glucosamine continued strong. At the end of eight weeks there was a big difference between the two groups. On a scale of 0 to 3, with 3 being the most painful, the glucosamine sulfate group had a pain score of 0.8 compared to 2.2 for the ibuprofen group. Additional swelling of the knee stopped in 20 percent of the glucosamine subjects and 0 percent in ibuprofen. Other studies confirm the results.

One study that involved 100 arthritis patients found 35 percent had adverse side effects with ibuprofen and only 6 percent in the glucosamine group. An Italian study looked at overall pain scales on a scale of 1 to 10, with 10 being more pain. The glucosamine group had a score of 2.4 compared to 8.3 for the placebo group after the study.

Overall, studies have found glucosamine sulfate to be both safe and effective by helping the body to repair eroded cartilage. It reduces pain, relieves swelling and tenderness, and has fewer side effects. When combined with chondroitin, the effects are even better.

Chondroitin

Chondroitin sulfate is another over the counter supplement that helps heal osteoarthritis. Chondroitin helps attract fluid into the proteoglycan molecule, the fluid serving as a spongy shock absorber attracting nutrients into the cartilage. Without this vital fluid, cartilage would become dry, malnourished, thinner, and more fragile. Other functions of chondroitin sulfate include:

1. Protects cartilage from premature damage.
2. Interferes with those enzymes that try to starve cartilage.
3. Stimulates the production of proteoglycans and collagen.
4. Works in cooperation with glucosamine sulfate.

Chondroitin sulfate supplements are nontoxic as shown in a six-year study of people taking 1.5 to 10 grams daily. An Italian study found osteoarthritis subjects had significantly less pain compared to a placebo group. A second Italian study found chondroitin sulfate provided pain relief and better mobility to osteoarthritis subjects compared to a control group. There were no side effects.

A French double blind study of 120 knee osteoarthritis patients compared one group who were given chondroitin to a placebo group. At the end of three months, the chondroitin group had significantly less pain and more function. A 1987 double blind study in Argentina compared a group of osteoarthritis subjects who were given chondroitin sulfate and aspirin to a group given a placebo and aspirin. Following 20 weeks, 13 of 17 subjects receiving chondroitin and aspirin had less pain compared to the control/placebo/aspirin group which had only 2 of 17 subjects reporting pain relief.

Most health food stores sell a supplement containing both glucosamine and chondroitin because they are more effective when taken together. The combination synthesizes new cartilage, while keeping the cartilage destroying enzyme under control. By normalizing the cartilage matrix, it essentially treats osteoarthritis at a cellular level. Dr. Theodosakis states that the combination of glucosamine and chondroitin "can stop osteoarthritis in its tracks and help heal the body." He believes the reasons most doctors don't use it is because of a mixture of conservatism, consumer's attitude, and commercial reality. In other words, drug companies cannot patent supplements to make big money, and so they do not research supplements such as chondroitin.

Super Flex

Super Flex is a pain reliving remedy that has been studied by researchers from Oxford University who consider it to be a new solution for joint pain. Over 100,000 pain sufferers have been helped by Super Flex.

Super Flex contains a natural plant enzyme called Bromelain known for its powerful anti-inflammatory and joint soothing ability. Clinical trials confirm "it is both safe and effective in achieving long-lasting pain relief without nasty side effects of traditional drugs." Oxford researchers studied 90 subjects with chronic pain and found after six weeks, Super Flex was as effective as popular prescription drugs. A Canadian study found a significant reduction in pain and swelling after 30 days. Another study involving 27 hospitals on 721 subjects found Super Flex reduced pain by an average of 73.7%.

Studies have found the active ingredient has been shown to break up fibrin by increasing plasmin enzyme levels, which reduces inflammation in joints. Scientists believe we feel more pain as we get older because our ability to produce enough plasmin to dissolve fibrin significantly decreases with age.

Super Flex stops joint pain, swelling, and irritation. Some consider it to be one of the most powerful natural pain relievers available. Call (800) 304-5530 to order Super Flex.

Exercise for Arthritis

Strong muscles are crucial for both preventing the onset of arthritis and for reducing symptoms. As people age, their muscle mass declines. After the age of 40 years, muscle mass decreases 1 percent a year, so by the age of 70, 30 percent of the muscle mass is lost compared to the age of 40. As a result, strength is also lost. This is why it is so important to be in an exercise program.

Yoga and Pilates

A comprehensive program of either yoga and Pilates is considered the most effective method for maximizing joint health. Because of various yoga postures, meditation and physical development have facilitated breathing so that every cell of the body benefits. Studies have shown that yoga is effective because its controlled breathing provides high levels of oxygen to nourish muscles, ligaments, and other tissues.

One of Hatha yoga's benefits is the practice of forceful breathing. If one breathes deeply into the lungs, this will activate the calming receptor found in the lung's lower lobe. For millennia, the calming effect of deep breathing has been known by the East. A 1994 study in the *Journal of Rheumatology* found that yoga significantly improved pain, tenderness, and range of motion of fingers in osteoarthritis patients. Another 1994 study was published in the *British Journal of Rheumatology* reporting yoga was beneficial for rheumatoid arthritis. Yoga has been found to benefit many ailments such as depression and chronic pain. It has been found to increase circulation and balance, and lowers cholesterol and improves the hormone system.

Joseph Pilates (1880-1967) founded the exercise of Pilates that utilizes yoga postures and controlled breathing as a starting point. He then added dynamic muscle work to each posture enhancing flexibility, strength, and endurance.

Tai Chi

Many rheumatologists and physical therapists recommend gentle exercise for patients with muscle and joint disease. One such exercise is tai chi, which is practiced in the East and balances and enhances the life energy of chi (qi). Traditional Chinese Medicine believes that disease is caused by a block or imbalance in the flow of qi through the body. Tai chi has been found to cure illness, strengthen organs, and improve the function of all body systems. Instructors of tai chi have found it effective for people with autoimmune disease including rheumatoid arthritis. Meditation and gentle soft movements are the cornerstones of tai chi. This exercise is described as part exercise, part martial arts, and part spiritual practice. Tai chi is a series of controlled movements that flow together in rhythm into one long graceful gesture. Movements are performed slowly and lightly, with concentration and inner stillness. Daily practice of tai chi is recommended.

Qigong

Qigong is another Eastern exercise which is a system of meditation and movement to strengthen and direct the flow of qi through the body to promote healing and self healing. Qigong movements are separate movements with each being held for a few seconds or longer. Many Chinese studies report the benefits of tai chi and gigong. Two studies in 1996 found tai chi and gigong significantly decreased the risk of falling for seniors.

Evidence has shown that when a strength training program is combined with proper dietary changes, arthritis symptoms often resolve themselves without medication or surgery. Most adults with osteoarthritis, rheumatoid arthritis, fibromyalgia, and lupus can benefit from exercise. The Center for Disease Control states that scientific studies show that participation in moderate intensity, low impact physical activity several times a week can relieve pain, improve function, and create a better mood without worsening symptoms or disease severity.

All forms of exercises including aerobic, muscle strengthening, and movement such as yoga and stretching promotes flexibility. Exercise keeps joints fully mobile while transporting nutrients to and from the cartilage to regulate and control swelling and pain. Exercise also promotes the quality of sleep and decreases fatigue. It enhances weight loss and promotes long-term weight management. Studies have found for every 10 pounds of excess weight, it takes one year off of life expectancy. The Framingham Study in the 1980s followed osteoarthritis patients for 35 years. The heaviest 20 percent of women had a seven times greater risk of developing knee arthritis compared to normal weight women.

Swimming is an excellent form of exercise for anyone suffering from arthritis and obesity. It is easy on the joints and excellent for the cardiovascular system while increasing muscle and bone strength. One should find an exercise they enjoy because it is easier to stick with such a program.

Dr. Vad lists arthritis friendly exercises in his book *Arthritis Rx* that include:

Safe Exercises
1. Aqua therapy
2. Swimming
3. Brisk walking
4. Bicycling
5. Low impact aerobic
6. Tai Chi
7. Qigong

Moderate Exercises
1. Golf
2. Cross country skiing
3. Softball
4. Elliptical training
5. Gardening with stool
6. Tennis
7. Yoga, Pilates

Unsafe Exercises
1. Jogging/running
2. StairMaster
3. Football
4. Soccer
5. Basketball
6. Hockey
7. Rock climbing

The cardinal rule for arthritis subjects is to never exercise through joint pain. A companion to exercise is good nutrition, which is also effective in relieving and eliminating pain, but first let's review several other types of arthritis.

Rheumatoid Arthritis

Rheumatoid arthritis is an autoimmune disease, meaning the body's immune system attacks the body's healthy tissue, specifically the synovium, the membrane that lines the joint. Some believe that rheumatoid arthritis is initiated by a bacterial infection or virus in the joints. Approximately two million people in the United States are affected by rheumatoid arthritis, with about 10 percent having a single episode that is followed by long-term remission. Aspirin and NSAIDs are the first line of therapy, and limited doses of corticosteroids are sometimes used. Surgery is an option in more severe cases. Numerous natural remedies have been found to be helpful according to scientific studies, many of them being herbs as discussed later in this chapter and in the nutrition chapter. Exercise has been found to reduce pain, joint stiffness and swelling.

Rheumatoid arthritis affects two to three times more women than men. About one half of rheumatoid arthritis sufferers are unable to work. At first, smaller joints are affected, especially fingers attached to hands and toes attached to feet. Then it can affect the larger body joints. There is no treatment or cure for the disease. Severe rheumatoid arthritis patients are at higher risk for infections, lung disease, heart failure, and heart attacks.

Gout

In 2011, more than 8 million Americans were affected by gout. Gout is the most common form of inflammation arthritis in men, affecting 3.4 million men. Gout is associated with obesity, insulin resistance, high blood pressure, and blood lipid issues. Individuals with gout either have a defect in eliminating uric acid or their body makes too much of it. Uric acid is formed by a breakdown of purines. As uric acid builds up in the blood, sharp crystals form that collect in the joints and soft tissue, resulting in inflammation and pain. Often the big toe is where gout attacks begin as well as the foot and ankle. Kidney stones are caused by high uric acid.

Gout can be controlled by reducing foods with high purines found in meat, poultry, dried beans, peas, scallops, sardines, cauliflower, and mushrooms. Both fasting and alcohol can raise uric acid levels. A gout sufferer should adopt a plant-based vegan diet and eliminate all animal-based food and processed foods. Cherries have been linked to a 35% lower risk of gout attacks. Research has shown tart cherry juice reduces uric acid by 25%. One should drink two to three glasses of water to help the body rid itself of uric acid. Losing weight is a must, and exercise helps prevent and reverse gout. Today gout can be cured by drugs such as allopurinol and probenecid.

Ankylosing Spondylitis

Another form of arthritis is ankylosing spondylitis, a rheumatic disease found most commonly in young men. The inflammation usually begins in the lower back and always involves the sacroiliac joints where the lower spine meets the pelvis, and can spread to the buttocks, thigh, and up to the chest.

Nutrition and Arthritis

Most types of arthritis involve inflammation that we have discussed in detail in another chapter. Much of this nutrition section is based on nutritionist Dr. Gary Null's book *Reverse Arthritis and Pain Naturally*. To prevent and alleviate arthritis, it is important to create and live an anti-inflammation lifestyle, which includes an anti-inflammation diet discussed in detail in the nutrition chapter. A summary includes:

1. *Omega 3 fatty acids* halt the inflammation process. Foods high in omega 3 fatty acids include green leafy vegetables, flax seeds, walnuts, chia seeds, grains, legumes, fruits, wild salmon, and cold water fish. It is best not to eat farm fish because they have high omega 6 fatty acids and contaminants.

2. *Avoid omega 6 fatty acids* that cause inflammation. Chronic inflammation leads to osteoarthritis, rheumatoid arthritis, and gout. These foods include dairy products and meat. All animal based diets have arachidonic acid which is in the omega 6 family.

3. *Reduce fat consumption*, especially trans fats, saturated fats, and polyunsaturated fats. Most fats can be made by the body except for omega 3 fatty acids and omega 6 fatty acids. These fatty acids need to be in a ratio (omega 6 to omega 3) of 1 to 1 or 4 to 1 at the most. Today's diet has a ratio of 10-20 to 1 (omega 6 to omega 3).

4. *Reduce oxidative stress:* Free radicals can cause damage to protein, lipids, DNA, and all components of the cell. Oxidative stress can initiate inflammation, and if chronic, can lead to arthritis. The main antioxidant in our body is glutathione. Broccoli, Brussels sprouts, cabbage, cauliflower, garlic, onions, avocados, asparagus, and walnuts are a good source of antioxidants that also promote glutathione production in the body.

5. *Reduce refined carbohydrates, sugar, salt, and artificial additives:* Refined food is deplete in nutrients. Without a diet rich in antioxidants and phytochemicals, our cells are subject to damage from free radicals leading to premature aging and arthritis.

6. *Eat a vegetarian or vegan diet:* Symptoms of osteoarthritis, rheumatoid arthritis, and gout can be alleviated and often reversed by a vegetarian or vegan diet. Antioxidants and foods such as fruits and vegetables lower arachidionic acid and can prevent inflammation. Diet is very important in healing and reversing gout.

With gout, one needs to avoid high purine foods such as meat and fish. Studies have shown in rheumatoid arthritis, animal protein and processed food damage the immune system. Research has found that a low-fat vegan diet relieves pain, tenderness, stiffness, and function.

7. *Eliminate pro-inflammatory foods:* Such foods include refined carbohydrates, wheat, gluten, dairy, meat, poultry, and shell fish. One should avoid caffeine, alcohol, sugar, artificial sweeteners, chemical preservatives, coloring agents, table salt, deep fried or toasted foods, and night shade vegetables.

8. *Beverages:* One should drink herbal teas, non-dairy milk such as almond, rice, or oat milk, filtered water and freshly squeezed organic fruits and vegetable juices. Do not drink soft drinks.

9. *Sweeteners:* Individuals should avoid artificial sweeteners. Use raw honey or natural fruit sweeteners.

10. *Oils*: Use extra virgin olive oil, grape seed oil, or sesame oil.

11. *Fruits*: Good anti-inflammatory fruits include grapes, apples, citrus, papaya, berries, and pomegranates.

12. *Herbs and spices:* Good spices include cayenne, curcumin, cinnamon, thyme, and chile pepper.

13. *Avoid high acid foods* such as refined sugar, flour, dairy, meat, seafood, soft drinks, coffee, and alcohol. All are associated with arthritis.

14. *Vegetables:* Studies have found many vegetables are beneficial for arthritis and inflammation including:
    A. *Alfalfa* inhibits cytokines involved with inflammation. Alfalfa relieves joint pain and reduces uric acid in joints.
    B. *Avugula* is anti-inflammatory and increases vitamin K.

C. *Asparagus* boosts immunity and reduces inflammation.
D. *Barley grass* has antioxidants that can relieve rheumatoid arthritis symptoms.
E. *Broccoli* helps heal both osteoarthritis and rheumatoid arthritis.
F. *Cabbage* is anti-inflammatory.
G. *Carrots* contains vitamin A, vitamin K, and carotenoid, which provide support for arthritis.
H. *Celery* has been used to treat arthritis for centuries.
I. *Collard greens* is a good anti-oxidant source that decreases oxidation and inflammation.
J. *Kale* is good against inflammation.
K. *Onions* reduce oxidative stress and inflammation.
L. *Parsley* is good against inflammation.
M. *Radishes* promote healing and modulate inflammation.
N. *Spinach* is anti-inflammatory.

15. *Fruits* are very beneficial for arthritis. Some of the best include:
    A. *Acai Berry* has been found in studies to relieve joint pain and benefit range of motion.
    B. *Bilberry* is a beneficial antioxidant that helps inflammation and stabilizes tendons, ligaments, and cartilage.
    C. *Blackberries* have the highest antioxidant activity of over 1,000 foods tested. It is high in vitamin C.
    D. *Blueberries* have good antioxidants that reduce inflammation.
    E. *Cherries* are anti-inflammatory, and in an osteoarthritis study significantly reduced pain and increased mobility.
    F. *Cranberries* are anti-inflammatory.

G. *Elderberries* boost immunity, are anti-inflammatory, and are good for arthritis.
H. *Guana* has powerful antioxidants that provides pain relief to inflammatory diseases.
I. *Kiwis* have antioxidants that protect DNA.
J. *Mango* has analgesic affects and antioxidant properties. Studies show it is anti-inflammatory.
K. *Mangosteen* has impressive anti-arthritic properties.
L. *Noni* studies found it is highly beneficial for arthritis sufferers.
M. *Oranges* are anti-inflammatory with studies showing an inverse relationship between consumption and arthritis.
N. *Pomegranate* studies have found it improves joint pain in rheumatoid arthritis.
O. *Papaya* is good for reducing inflammation and has been used to treat arthritis around the world.
P. *Pineapple* contains bromelain that suppress inflammation and moderates joint pain.
Q. *Prunes* reduce oxidative stress.
R. *Pumpkins* have high anti-oxidant properties that reduce inflammation.
S. *Raspberries* contain a high content of ellagic acid and anthrocyanin that limit inflammation and relieve pain.
T. *Strawberries* contain many antioxidants that are anti-inflammatory.
U. *Watermelon* reduces oxidative stress and inflammation.

16. Other Nutrients
    A. *Chia seeds* are good for fighting arthritis.
    B. *Chlorella* is a type of algae that reduces DNA oxidation. Studies show it helps prevent and treat arthritis.

C. *Coconut oil* has a natural form of saturated fat that boosts immunity; it is anti-inflammatory, and relieves pain.
D. *Flaxseed* has high levels of omega 3 fatty acids. A meta-analysis of a number of studies found it is a beneficial treatment for joint pain associated with rheumatoid arthritis.
E. *Garlic* has abundant anti-inflammatory sulfur compounds which fight arthritis. One study found 86 percent of rheumatoid patients had a good response.
F. *Ginger root* contain antioxidants called gingerols effective in treating animal rheumatoid arthritis.
G. *Green tea* has a number of compounds that promote joint health and helps with a variety of arthritis types.
H. *Spirulina* is blue green algae that decreases inflammation related to arthritis in mice studies. It helped mice recover.
I. *Vinegar and honey* is an old time remedy for arthritis. Mix a tablespoon of apple cider vinegar with a tablespoon of honey and stir them into a warm glass of water. Drink this mixture two to three times a day.

Supplements for Arthritis

Supplements are discussed in more detail in the nutrition chapter. Follow Dr. Null's protocol on how to take supplements found in that chapter.

A. *Bromelain* is an enzyme derived from pineapple. It relieves pain and improves physical mobility. The dose depends on the pain level.
B. *Chondroitin* helps heal joint cartilage. (1,200 mg).
C. *Decursinol* is in a class called coumarin that relieves pain and protects against oxidative stress.

D. *Gamma Linolenic Acid (GLA)* is high in prostaglandins that turns off inflammation plus reducing pain. (240 mg daily)
E. *Glucosamine* repairs joint cartilage and tissue damage. (1,500 – 2,000 mg daily)
F. *Grape seed extract* contains pycnogen, which is an antioxidant that strengthens collagen. (100 mg daily)
G. *Hyaluronic Acid* is found in abundance in joint tissue. (200 mg daily)
H. *Methylsulfonylmethane (MSM)* suppresses inflammation and reduces pain. (500 mg daily)
I. *Minerals*: Beneficial minerals for arthritis include calcium, phosphorous, boron, magnesium, zinc, selenium, potassium, copper, and manganese. Many of these minerals may be in your multivitamin supplement. Take daily.
J. *Niacinamide* will reduce arthritis symptoms and improve range of motion. (150 - 250 mg before meals, 3 or 4 times daily)
K. *Omega 3 fatty acids* are anti-inflammatory and relieve pain. (2,000 mg daily)
L. *Probiotic* is a beneficial bacteria supplement for digestion and immunity.
M. *Quercetin* is a naturally occurring flavonoid that is an antioxidant and immune booster. (500 mg daily)
O. *S-adenosyl-L-methionine (SAMe)* restores white blood cell activity in joint fluid and reverses glutathione depletion. It protects and rebuilds cartilage. (400 mg daily)
P. *Superoxide dismutase (SOD)* provides arthritis relief with vitamin E. (2,000 mg daily)
Q. *Vitamin B complex* regulates nervous system health and utilization of other nutrients.
R. *Vitamin K* is a potent anti-inflammatory vitamin that helps and treats arthritis. (2 mg daily)

S. *Zingerflex* contains 1500 mg glucosamine, 1200 mg chondroitin sulfate, and 510 mg of ginger. (4 capsules daily)

Herbs for Arthritis

A number of herbs have been effective for arthritis. They are discussed in detail in the nutrition chapter. For more information, refer to that chapter. The following is a summary.

A. *Aloe Vera* cleans the body of toxins that are associated with arthritis. (Drink 2 ounces of aloe vera juice twice daily)
B. *Boswellia* is an anti-inflammatory Ayurvedic medicine herb that is effective for arthritis. (100 mg daily)
C. *Cat's Claw* is an anti-inflammatory herb with studies showing it is effective in osteoarthritis.
D. *Cayenne* comes from cayenne pepper containing capsaicin which reduces arthritis pain. The cream helps both osteoarthritis and rheumatoid arthritis. (50 mg of cayenne twice daily)
E. *Comfrey* has been shown in studies to relieve pain and improve mobility in arthritis patients.
F. *Devil's Claw* is an herb that has been used for centuries to relieve pain. Studies show it is anti-arthritic with analgesic properties. (100 mg daily)
G. *Ginseng* is an anti-inflammatory herb that stimulates the immune system.
H. *Nettles* is a plant that has anti-inflammatory properties for osteoarthritis and rheumatoid arthritis.
I. *Turmeric* is a natural anti-inflammatory herb that reduces joint pain, stiffness, and improves mobility.
J. *White willow bark* is a powerful analgesic for people suffering from joint pain. This is where aspirin originated. (400 mg daily)

Amniotic Stem Cell Therapy

Stem cell therapy may be the next big health care advancement in non-surgical pain management. Many consider it to be the medicine of the future. The procedure for amniotic stem cell therapy for pain was discovered in 2007, and research began in 2011 to explore its many potentials for pain management and other attributes.

Stem cells are natural cells found in the body that are responsible for healing damaged joints, cartilage, and muscles. The body is constantly rebuilding the damaged tissue with the help of stem cells. After the age of 40, the number of stem cells and their potency significantly decrease each year. This explains why a 21-year-old person can heal much faster than a 65-year-old.

Stem cells used at pain clinics are called "amniotic stem cells," which come from the amniotic sac, not from embryos. Amniotic stem cells are harvested from a donating mother during a scheduled c-section, and then processed at an FDA approved lab. The cells are rigorously tested like other biological tissue before they are sent to pain clinics. The use of amniotic stem cells raises no moral issues, unlike embryo stem cells. Amniotic stem cells are 'neutral cells' that contain no DNA. Because of this neutrality, patients cannot have a rejection or reaction to them. They are completely safe. Since 2007, there has not been one adverse effect documented in the tens of thousand procedures.

Amniotic stem cells can turn into almost any type of tissue because they just grew a baby. They are brand new cells which are extremely potent, meaning they can heal tissue very quickly in most parts of the body. For example, a patient may have meniscus damage in the joint, a frayed ligament, weak tendons, and minor fracture of the bone. Amniotic stem cells have the ability to heal all those structures.

Amniotic stem cells are reported to have natural anti-inflammatory and pain relieving properties that are more effective than steroids. Pain clinics report the majority of patients leave the clinic with little or no pain by the time the analgesic wears off. For example, knee tissue has healed enough so there is no longer pain.

A pain-score study conducted on 200 patients at the Pain MD Clinic in Coeur d'Alene, Idaho found that before treatment, the average pain score was 7.7 on a scale of one to ten. After one month, the average pain score was 3.1. After 27 months, the clinical improvement held. In 95% of the cases, only one procedure was required. The results are even better when combined with Platelet Rich Plasma Therapy.

The procedure takes less than 20 minutes, which involves injection into the painful area. It often heals other parts of the body. Clinical findings have found amniotic stem cell therapy is effective for osteoarthritis, rheumatoid arthritis, back pain, neuropathy, fibromyalgia, erectile dysfunction, Alzheimer's disease, Parkinson's disease, multiple sclerosis, thyroid conditions, cancer, visual disturbances, macular degeneration, and many more conditions.

Stem cell therapy has been effective for diabetic neuropathy because it can grow new blood vessels and nerves. Relief comes in four weeks. There have been 45 clinical studies involving 1,272 patients. It prevents amputation.

At this time insurance companies and medicare do not cover stem cell therapy. The price at the Pain MD Clinic in Coeur d'Alene, Idaho is about $6,500. For a free consultation call (208) 667-7246. Their website is www.idpainmd.com. Another stem cell clinic for pain is located in northern Colorado at the Premier Stem Cell Institute. Call (866) 647-9405 for a free consultation.

The next chapter will discuss another form of arthritis, fibromyalgia, that encompasses both pain and fatigue.

Chapter Seven

Fibromyalgia

Pain and Fatigue

The fibromyalgia syndrome has appeared only recently on the scene, recognized in 1987 by the American Medical Association as a disorder. In 1990, the American College of Rheumatology gave it a definition. The Center for Disease Control and Prevention estimated 5 million Americans suffered from fibromyalgia in 2005 as reported in the journal *Arthritis and Rheumatology*. Other sources state that 2 percent of the adult population in the United States suffer from fibromyalgia with similar distributions in other countries. Adult women are affected 5 to 7 times more commonly than men. Much of the information in this chapter comes from an excellent book entitled *Fibromyalgia Syndrome, A Practitioners Guide to Treatment* written by Dr. Leon Chaitow, an osteopath and naturopath.

What is fibromyalgia? The American College of Rheumatology defines it as a history of widespread pain for at least three years. A diagnosis consists of identifying 11 of 18 tender point sites upon digital pressure. Fibromyalgia is a non-deforming rheumatic condition that has no cause or cure. The term rheumatic can be defined as a painful but non-deforming soft tissue musculoskeletal condition. The problem with the American College of Rheumatology's definition is that research shows that 20 percent of the population suffers widespread pain but do not demonstrate all 11 of 18 tender points. So what diagnosis is appropriate for this group?

Professor Stephen Stahl, from the University of California San Diego, in his book *Chronic Pain and Fibromyalgia,* describes fibromyalgia as having chronic widespread pain associated with fatigue, altered mood, and cognitive problems. Dr. Stahl does not think the 11 tender points are the most accurate criteria to diagnose fibromyalgia. The cause is unknown, but fibromyalgia is closely related to depression and anxiety. The higher the number of painful symptoms, the greater the likelihood that a patient has a mood or anxiety disorder. Cognitive symptoms that accompany fibromyalgia may often include a 'foggy' mind, memory problems, forgetfulness, a blurring of mental activities, sensory overload, and a decreased ability to process information. There are a number of hypotheses that try to explain the cause of fibromyalgia.

Theories on the Cause of Fibromyalgia

1. *Abnormal Neurochemical Process*

   Nearly three decades of research has produced no single pattern that sheds light on the cause of fibromyalgia. There is growing evidence that an abnormal neurochemical process is occurring to the sensory signals going to the central nervous system. This results in a lowering of the pain threshold causing an amplification of normal sensory signals that result in patients experiencing constant pain.

2. *Allergies*

   Some evidence suggests that allergies may be linked to both fibromyalgia and chronic fatigue. Particular foods or substances can be shown to provoke or exacerbate pain and fatigue in fibromyalgia. So what causes food allergies? Often it is initiated by malabsorption of large molecules through the intestinal wall. This may have resulted from yeast and bacterial overgrowth resulting from antibiotics and disturbances of the normal flora. Some suggest it may be gluten sensitivity from wheat. Allergies can aggravate pain.

3. *Genetics*

   Evidence suggests there is certainly more than one form of fibromyalgia, with some people having a genetic predisposition triggered by a single traumatic experience, either physical or psychological. It may be an infection, or perhaps a toxic overload that triggers it. One study found that 43 percent of 42 fibromyalgia patients had joint hypermobility, which is a genetic acquired trait. Mitral valve prolapse was found in 75 percent of fibromyalgia patients in one study, again suggesting a possible genetic connection.

4. *Immune Dysfunction*

   Some researchers believe fibromyalgia may be due to an immune dysfunction. The immune system seems to be provoked into an excessive response resulting in elevated cytokine production found in fibromyalgia patients. This potentiates allergy symptoms, reduces blood flow to the brain, and disturbs brain function. The hypothalamus is disturbed which causes sleep problems, digestive problems, and hormone imbalance. The immune dysfunction could be triggered by a viral infection, stress, or trauma resulting in increased cytokine production leading to brain dysfunction. As a consequence, serotonin receptors in the brain can be modified which influences sleep, temper, mood, fatigue, and pain tolerance.

5. *Stress Hormones*

   Another hypothesis involves stress hormones, specifically cortisol. Studies show lower than normal cortisol levels in fibromyalgia patients. Some studies conclude that patients with fibromyalgia have an impaired ability to activate the hypothalamus-pituitary-adrenal axis (HPA axis). As a result, the adrenal glands that secrete cortisol are hypoactive. Another study concluded that psychological factors and the HPA axis could explain the pain variance in fibromyalgia patients. Cortisol is produced in response to most stress events including infection, inflammation, trauma, and emotional stress. Cortisol deficiencies are characterized by fatigue, weakness, muscle joint pain, and irritable bowel syndrome.

6. *Hypothyroidism*

    A hypothesis involving a dysfunctional thyroid gland may provide light on the cause of fibromyalgia. The symptoms of fibromyalgia closely resemble those of hypothyroidism, which include depression, mental fatigue, anxiety, poor memory, sleep disturbance, gastro-intestinal dysfunction, fatigue, low body temperature, and musculoskeletal symptoms. Fibromyalgia is often a diagnosis for hypothyroidism. Several studies have been conducted involving thyroid medication for fibromyalgia without side effects. Thyroid hormones regulate substance P which is high in fibromyalgia patients. Some researchers conclude that inadequate regulation of gene transcription by thyroid hormones could not only account for high substance P but for all other objective findings and associated symptoms of fibromyalgia.

7. *Sleep Disorders*

    Disturbed sleep leads to reduced serotonin production, with a consequent reduction in pain modulation effect of endorphins and increased substance P.

8. *Muscle Microtrauma and Growth Hormone*

    Muscle microtrauma due to a genetic predisposition or to growth hormone dysfunction can lead to calcium leakage and increasing muscle contraction that reduces the oxygen supply. This can lead to a decrease in mitochondrial energy resulting in fatigue and pain.

9. *Pain Modulation Disorder*

    Fibromyalgia may be a pain modulation disorder resulting from brain dysfunction in the limbic area that leads to mistranslation of sensory signals.

10. *Toxicity etc.*

    Some researchers believe that fibromyalgia may be a combination of toxins, allergies, infection, and nutrition deficiencies that produce symptoms.

11. *Blood Type*
    Fibromyalgia conditions may be related to blood type intolerance, specifically type O blood, resulting from an interaction between food derived lectins and specific tissue related to blood type.

12. *Hyperventilation*
    Many fibromyalgia patients demonstrate low carbon dioxide levels when resting, suggesting possible hyperventilation. Symptoms of hyperventilation closely mimic fibromyalgia. Hyperventilation stresses the muscles of the upper body and produces oxygen deprivation in the brain.

13. *Emotions*
    Called psychogenic rheumatism, fibromyalgia may be caused by emotions that directly impact pain perception and immune function.

14. *Myofascial Pain Syndrome*
    Fibromyalgia is thought by some to be an extreme form of myofascial pain syndrome.

15. *Body Trauma*
    Body trauma such as whiplash from an auto accident seems to be an important factor in triggering the onset of fibromyalgia.

16. *Virus*
    Some scientists think it may be a virus or other microbe trigger that leads to an overactive immune system. Chemical sensitivities, food allergies, hypothalamus disturbances, and hormone imbalance may also cause overactivation.

Triggers for Fibromyalgia Pain

Fibromyalgia is a chronic painful musculoskeletal condition characterized by widespread aching points of tenderness. Neural structures can become hyper reactive in either spinal or paraspinal tissue. When change occurs in ligaments, tendons, or periosteal tissue, they are called trigger points. If located in muscles, they are called myofascial trigger points. Any form of stress, be it climate, toxic, emotional, or physical will produce neurological output from the trigger point.

Emotional arousal affects the susceptibility of neural pathways for these triggers. In chronic pain settings, non-pain neurons can be sensitized to carry pain impulses. This hyper-sensitization of spinal nerves may involve non-pain neurons that are altered which lead to increased levels of substance P in the cerebral spinal fluid. Because of this hypersensitivity, these non-pain neurons register pain which would otherwise be a benign impulse. Localized areas of neural facilitation can occur in almost all soft tissue called myofascial trigger points. Therefore the pain in fibromyalgia is exaggerated in all forms of stress. The following factors can enhance myofascial trigger points.

1. Nutritional deficiency, especially vitamin C, B complex, and iron
2. Hormone deficiencies such as low thyroid production, menopause, or premenstrual syndrome (PMS)
3. Infections caused by viruses, bacteria, or yeasts
4. Allergies, especially wheat (gluten) and dairy
5. Low oxygen to tissue caused by tension, stress, inactivity, or poor respiration

Myofascial trigger points are not the cause of fibromyalgia but do contribute to the pain aspect. There are a number of ways to deactivate and modulate myofascial trigger points, including microcurrent or electro-acupuncture.

Symptoms of Fibromyalgia

Pain and fatigue are hallmark symptoms of fibromyalgia. A number of conditions are associated with fibromyalgia raising the question if these conditions are the cause or effect. Following is a list of conditions accompanying fibromyalgia compared to the general population:

Condition	% in Fibromyalgia	% in General population
Chronic Headaches	50	5
Dysmenorrhea	60	15
Endometriosis	15	2
Interstitial Cystitis	25	<1
Irritable Bladder/ Urethral Pain	15	<1
Irritable Bowel Syndrome	68	10
Mitral Valve Prolapse	75	15
Multiple Chemical Sensitivities	40	5
Restless Leg Syndrome	30	2
Temporal Mandibular Joint Disorder	25	5

A study conducted on 280 fibromyalgia patients, which included 97 percent women, found they had preexisting conditions of arthritis (65%), depression (62%), irritable bowel syndrome (52%), temporal joint disorder (41%), carpel tunnel syndrome (30%), hypothyroid (24%), panic attacks (23%), blood sugar imbalance (19%), cancer (9%), Raynaud syndrome (7%), and eating disorders (3%).

Before contracting fibromyalgia syndrome, 62% reported physical or emotional trauma, 46% reported adverse drug reactions, 43% reported fever blisters, 24% had close contact with toxic materials, 21% had feverish episodes, 20% reported mononucleosis, 9% contracted herpes, and 6% received breast implants.

Symptoms associated with fibromyalgia in the study of the 280 patients included:

1. Affected by cold and damp weather 83%

2. Poor sleep patterns 82%

3. Tired easily 81%

4. Spinal problems 81%

5. Used over the counter medication 78%

6. Sensitive to cold 68%
7. Allergies 67%
8. Frequent headaches 65%
9. Trouble controlling bladder 61%
10. Difficulty communicating feelings 59%
11. Pelvic pain, urinary urgency 58%
12. Light headed 57%
13. Premenstrual syndrome 56%

Another study examined 1,000 fibromyalgia and chronic fatigue patients regarding their symptoms, which included:

1. Chronic fatigue 100%
2. Cold extremities 100%
3. Impaired memory 100%
4. Frequent urination 95%
5. Depression 94%
6. Sleep disorders 94%
7. Balance problems 89%
8. Muscle twitching 80%
9. Dry mouth 68%
10. Muscle aches 68%
11. Headaches 68%
12. Sore throat 20%

Common Signs
1. Elevated body temperature 10%
2. Normal temperature 25%
3. Low body temperature 65%
4. Yeast infection 87%
5. Tender thyroid 40%
6. White spots on ovaries 85%
7. Fibromyalgia tender spots 81%
8. Abdominal tenderness 80%
9. Swollen lymph nodes 18%

Lab Findings
1. Yeast in stools 82%
2. Parasites in stools 30%
3. Magnesium deficiency 38%
4. Zinc deficiency 32%

Symptoms Before Onset
1. Irritable bowel syndrome 89%
2. Constant gas/bloating 80%
3. Constipation 58%
4. Recurrent sinusitis 30%
5. Bladder infection 20%
6. Premenstrual syndrome 90%
7. Endometriosis 65%
8. Anxiety disorder 22%
9. Sleep disorder 1%

Associated Conditions of Fibromyalgia
1. Chronic myofascial pain in all patients.
2. Chronic fatigue syndrome is experienced by almost all fibromyalgia patients, with a greater emphasis on fatigue than pain.
3. Multiple chemical sensitivity is found in many fibromyalgia patients.
4. Post traumatic stress disorder is a common condition.

One common feature in all the above listed conditions is based on the toxic/biochemical hypothesis that involves elevated levels of nitric oxide and its potent oxidant product peroxynitrate.

The Mind and Fibromyalgia

As in most health disorders, the mind plays a vital role in both the cause and symptoms of fibromyalgia. Studies have shown the pathophysiology of fibromyalgia involves a complex relationship with stress and its impact on physiological pathways involving pain and cognition. Research shows fibromyalgia patients suffer three times higher rates of mental disorders compared to subjects without pain. Depression can help predict the onset of pain symptoms among pain-free subjects.

Early Life Events
A considerable amount of evidence suggests that adverse early-life events such as neglect, physical abuse, or sexual abuse are associated with chronic pain in adulthood. Women with fibromyalgia are significantly more likely to report rape, sexual abuse, and physical abuse both in childhood and adulthood. Childhood abuse has been identified as a trigger to fibromyalgia as has emotional stress. Many fibromyalgia patients also experience lifelong victimization.

One study found that fibromyalgia patients reported poor relationships with their mother, and even poorer relationships with their father. They generally felt less secure compared to other pain patients. For fibromyalgia patients who report the greatest level of childhood adversity, it is often followed by a somatic form-pain disorder. Other research has found prior to the age of 16, many fibromyalgia patients report a series of events such as an ill parent, separation or death of a parent, a hospital operation, or abuse when compared to a control group without fibromyalgia.

Stressors

Widespread pain disorders, including fibromyalgia, are common symptoms of traumatic road traffic accidents. Other stressors associated with fibromyalgia are workplace injuries, military deployment, chronic viral infections such as Lyme disease, dietary toxins, and environmental chemicals. Also associated with fibromyalgia are a patient's mindset regarding hypochondrial beliefs, hyper-vigilance to pain, increased pain-related fear, reduced pain threshold, increased psychological distress, and poor pain coping.

Studies have found those suffering from chronic fatigue syndrome and fibromyalgia have three overlapping psychological factors including depression, anxiety, and poor stress coping skills. Some researchers believe fibromyalgia may be caused by emotions that impact pain perception and immune function. Highly emotional people show a higher incidence of local areas of myofascial distress, such as pain, because emotions are able to affect the susceptibility of neural pathways to sensitization.

Depression

Sixty-two percent of fibromyalgia patients suffered from depression before their diagnosis. Once diagnosed with fibromyalgia, 94 percent experience depression, 100 percent have impaired memory, and another 94 percent suffer from sleep disorders. Some researchers wonder if fibromyalgia is a form of depression because there are so many similar symptoms between the two disorders. Depression and fibromyalgia patients demonstrate similar responses to psychological scales. Both disorders have a high lifetime rate for mood disorders. Scientific evidence shows that mild antidepressant medication aids in symptom relief for fibromyalgia patients.

Studies have shown a greater family history of depression in fibromyalgia patients compared to rheumatoid arthritis patients and to a control group. Their history also showed a greater lifetime level of stress. Fortunately, most patients with fibromyalgia do not have psychiatric illness. Still the question is asked, is depression the result of pain or is pain a result of depression? One study did conclude that fibromyalgia is not a condition of psychogenic origin.

Anxiety and Hyperventilation

Anxiety testing conducted on fibromyalgia patients suggest that the current anxiety they suffer is not secondary to pain but actually may be causing it. A common symptom of fibromyalgia is over-breathing (hyperventilation) which is common with anxiety. Anxious people tend to breathe dysfunctionally, involving the upper chest with minimal diaphragm movement. These breathing patterns can exacerbate both fibromyalgia and chronic fatigue. Breath retraining can reduce the effect of hyperventilation and minimize symptoms of fibromyalgia. Many researchers believe anxiety is a trigger to fibromyalgia, not a cause. Improper breathing can lead to ischemia, pain, and fatigue.

Sleep Disorders

Fibromyalgia is characterized by abnormal sleep in nearly all patients. Sleep disturbance can lead to reduced protein synthesis, decreased hormone secretion, and an upset hypo-thalamus/pituitary axis as found in fibromyalgia patients. Sleep disturbance (non-restorative sleep) is the most common symptom of fibromyalgia besides pain and fatigue. Disturbance in sleep is associated with greater pain and more severe symptoms. There are two reasons why sleep disturbance increases muscle pain. The first is a disruption of tissue repair resulting from a growth hormone deficit. The other reason is a decrease in interleukin 1, which is part of the immune modulation role of sleep. Antidepressant medication used by fibromyalgia is mainly used to enhance sleep patterns. Insomnia in chronic pain is the same type as primary insomnia.

Fibromyalgia patients usually wake up feeling awful, with their optimal functioning occurring between 10:00 A.M. and 2:00 P.M. This disturbed sleep syndrome emerges from central nervous disturbance due to altered metabolic functions that affect serotonin, substance P, interleukin 1, growth hormone, and cortisol. All these biochemical changes contribute to the symptoms of fibromyalgia.

Chronic Fatigue

Chronic fatigue is a symptom experienced by over 90 percent of all fibromyalgia patients. Scientists believe it is a disorder involving the central nervous system due to altered permeability of the blood brain barrier. Factors that compromise the blood brain barrier include viruses, certain cytokines, nitric oxide, stress, glutathione depletion, essential fatty acid deficiencies, and toxins such as mercury. Some believe that the breakdown of the blood brain barrier disrupts neural transmission.

Researchers hypothesize that low serotonin and high substance P in the brain and spinal cord can lead to neural functional abnormalities including sleep disturbances, increased pain perception, and dysfunctional bowel symptoms. Substance P is elevated in fibromyalgia and is normally released by the spinal cord in response to pain. Serotonin inhibits neurotransmitters necessary for maintaining restorative sleep and acts on the thalamus gland to regulate pain perception. Low serotonin is found in fibromyalgia patients.

Chronic fatigue syndrome and fibromyalgia have similar clinical characteristics, no known cause, no effective therapy, and both are chronic. About 70 percent of chronic fatigue patients meet the diagnostic criterion of fibromyalgia. Fibromyalgia is characterized by pain and chronic fatigue. Both involve elevated levels of nitrous oxide and its potent oxidant product peroxynitrate. Someone with fibromyalgia would qualify for a chronic fatigue diagnosis and a chronic fatigue syndrome patient with muscle and joint pain would fit a fibromyalgia diagnosis.

Therapies for Fibromyalgia

Fibromyalgic patients are difficult to treat and both patient and doctor often become frustrated by traditional therapy because of the complex nature of the disorder. Many patients find their best results from alternative therapies that we will explore along with traditional therapies. Often it means a committed lifestyle change. One study conducted on fibromyalgia patients asked what therapy worked best for their fibromyalgia. The results are as follows:

1. Pain Medication 67%
2. Help with Sleep Patterns 66%
3. Thermal Treatment 62%
4. Physical Exercise 61%
5. Antidepressant Medicine 60%
6. Hydro Therapy 51%
7. Physical Therapy 40%

Another study on 6,000 fibromyalgia/chronic fatigue syndrome patients looked at various attributes of both disorders.

A. *Known Triggers*
1. Physical Trauma 39%
2. Major Emotional Trauma 27%
3. Infection 20%
4. Surgery 9%
5. Exposure to Chemical Agent 5%

B. *Status after Therapy*
1. Fully Recovered 0.2%
2. Experienced Improvement 31%
3. Unchanged 20%
4. Worse 40%
5. Disabled 9%

C. *Associated Symptoms*
1. Memory and Concentration Difficulty 86%
2. Discomfort Following Exertion 89%
3. Waking Tired in the Morning 89%

Fibromyalgia

    4. Unable to work 40%
    5. Percent of Time in Pain 76%
    6. Percent of Body in Pain 71%

D. *Patient Satisfaction*
    1. Rheumatologist 51%
    2. Physical Therapy 13%
    3. Neurologist 10%
    4. Chiropractor 6%
    5. Internist 27%
    6. Family Physician 46%

E. *What Helped the Most on a Scale of 1 to 10?*
    1. Drugs and Non-Drug Therapy 4.8
    2. Educational Material 7.4

Traditional Therapy

Drugs

    Dawn Marcus, M.D., in her book *Chronic Pain: A Primary Care Guide* writes that fibromyalgia patients need to be reassured that fibromyalgia is not a disease, but a symptom complex. She states that symptoms are not progressive and will not lead to loss of muscle strength. Most patients will improve over time, with one study finding both pain and medication decreased over three years.

    Most studies regarding fibromyalgia have evaluated antidepressants, which effectively reduce fibromyalgia symptoms. The studies found there is only a modest superiority of antidepressants over a placebo, with short term effect better than long term effect.

    Tricyclic antidepressants (TCA) have been the most widely studied antidepressants for fibromyalgia. TCAs inhibit the reuptake of serotonin and are effective because fibromyalgia patients have low serotonin. Gabapentin is an anti-epileptic drug that benefits fibromyalgia patients. It can reduce pain, improve sleep, and reduce anxiety symptoms.

Tiznidine has been found to relieve pain, help muscle spasms, and improve sleep. Analgesics have limited benefit for fibromyalgia patients. Four studies found NSAID drugs are not superior to a placebo. Dr. Marcus claims fibromyalgia patients benefit greatly from education about their condition.

The Thyroid

We have discussed the association between fibromyalgia and hypothyroidism. Perhaps hypothyroidism is being under diagnosed. Broda Barnes, M.D., specialized in hypothyroidism during the last century in Fort Collins, Colorado and wrote a book entitled *Hypothyroidism* about his experience treating the disorder. Patients were coming world-wide to be treated by him. Dr. Barnes found that blood testing for hypothyroidism is not the best test for making a diagnosis. His diagnosis is based on basal body temperature, not blood thyroid tests. He believes so many people are being under diagnosed. If a patient has a basal body temperature below 98.6 degrees and has cold extremities, the patient is probably suffering from hypothyroidism even if the thyroid blood tests showed normal. Barnes then prescribed thyroid medications to raise the body temperature. By doing this, most of the patient's symptoms would disappear. Today, most physicians would not prescribe thyroid medication based on low basal body temperature. Most fibromyalgia patients have a low basal body temperature, so it might be worth consulting an open-minded physician to see if thyroid hormone would reduce fibromyalgia symptoms.

Dr. Leon Chaitow in his book *Fibromyalgia Syndrome* summarized most of the traditional and alternative treatments that have been effective for fibromyalgia. He also discusses thyroid therapy. His therapy involves either desiccated thyroid or T3 thyroid hormone. According to tissue response, Dr. Chaitow will adjust the dosage. He then instructs the patient to engage in activities that would capitalize on the increased capacity of the thyroid hormone.

A patient with primary or central hypothyroidism begins treatment with desiccated thyroid or T3 thyroid hormone. If the

Fibromyalgia

patient does not respond to T3, the physician increases the dosage and provides the patient with 20 mg of propranolol tablets to use only in case of overstimulation of the thyroid. Propranolol blocks the effect of thyroid hormone.

Most fibromyalgia patients start with 75 mcg of T3 or 60 mg of desiccated thyroid. Dosage is increased at one to two weeks with T3 and three to four weeks with desiccated thyroid. Dosage increases are 12.5 to 25 mcg of T3 or 30 to 60 mg of desiccated thyroid. It may take several weeks before the effect of an increase can be seen.

An electrocardiogram before each dosage adjustment can assure patient safety in terms of cardiac function. For patients that have rapid pounding of the heart with minimal exertion, they should have an ECG. If patients have a compromised cardiac function, the initial dosage should be low. Middle aged and elderly patients who are not in good physical condition should begin thyroid therapy at a low dosage. Dosage adjustments are made on the basis of peripheral measurements such as achilles reflex, serum cholesterol, and increased voltage of the ECG. The objective dosage adjustment is maximum improvement of all facets of fibromyalgia status.

The use of both thyroid and tricyclic antidepressants can cause a greater increase in heart rate than either medication taken alone. In some patients with treatment-resistant trigger points, they often respond to T3 treatment.

If one undergoes thyroid hormone therapy, the patient needs to engage in regular toning and aerobic exercise plus nutritional supplements. Mild hypoglycemia and low blood sugar become more severe when patients begin thyroid hormone therapy. Thyroid hormone increases the rate of glucose absorption from the GI tract.

Nutritional supplements that Dr. Chaitow recommends for fibromyalgia patients include:

1. Vitamin B complex   50-100 mg

2. Vitamin C   2,000-10,000 mg

3. Calcium   200 mg

4. Magnesium   1,000 mg

5. Multivitamins
6. Vitamin E 800 IU
7. Beta Carotene 30-90 mg

Medications
1. Tricyclic antidepressants have been effective with fibromyalgia.
2. Amitriptyline improved symptoms in 77 percent of fibromyalgia patients after five weeks.
3. Prozac is an antidepressant that can improve fibromyalgia symptoms.
4. Prozac plus Elevil taken daily have good results with fibromyalgia.

Alternative Treatments

Massage

Both massage and spinal manipulation seem to help many fibromyalgia patients. The goal is to increase circulation through the involved muscle region. Massage helps patients learn how to control pain through relaxation. A controlled study utilizing Swedish massage on fibromyalgia patients found it improved symptoms of pain, fatigue, anxiety, and depression compared to the control. With most fibromyalgia patients, the therapist should not do deep work.

Chiropractic

Fibromyalgia patients seem to benefit from spinal manipulation as much as they do from soft treatment of massage. Two controlled studies have shown spinal manipulation increases the overall well being of fibromyalgia patients. One study found 46 percent reported a moderate to a great deal of improvement from chiropractic therapy. Spinal manipulation is thought to release endogenous opioids (endorphins). Increased spinal mobility tends to decrease transmission of pain from adjacent structures.

Candida Infection

Many fibromyalgia patients have candida yeast over-growth, with symptoms of candida resembling fibromyalgia. Patients may have both conditions. Patients can help eliminate candida by changing the diet, avoiding corticosteroids, and not utilizing antibiotics.

Hypnotherapy

For patients not responding well to other forms of treatment, one study found hypnotherapy helped more than physical therapy for patients diagnosed with fibromyalgia.

Group Therapy

After six months, one study found when interdisciplinary therapies are used in group fibromyalgia treatment, 70 percent had reduced their number of tender points to fewer than the criterion used for diagnosing fibromyalgia.

Biofeedback

Several studies have suggested that fibromyalgia patients can benefit from mind body therapies. Improvement in tender points, pain intensity, and morning stiffness are helped by biofeedback.

Amniotic Stem Cell Therapy

Stem cells are natural cells found in the body that are responsible for healing damaged joints, cartilage, and muscles. Stem cell therapy may be the medicine of the future. Early clinical evidence suggests it helps with fibromyalgia. For more details, refer to Chapter Six on arthritis, regarding stem cell therapy.

Nutrition Supplements

1. **Thiamine** may be impaired in fibromyalgia patients. One study found injections of thiamine three times a week for six weeks gave relief to 95 percent of fibromyalgia patients.

2. **Magnesium** deficiency causes similar symptoms as fibromyalgia, such as muscle pain, fatigue, depression, sleep disorders, and anxiety. Fibromyalgia patients have significantly higher blood levels of calcium and magnesium, suggesting higher levels of secretion.
3. **Selenium** deficiencies may be associated with muscle pain. One study showed 60 percent of fibromyalgia patients benefitted when given selenium. When selenium was combined with vitamin E, the results were even better.
4. **Arginine** is an amino acid that helps pain and fatigue. Do not take longer than two to three months.
5. **S-adenosyl-L-methionine** reduces muscle tenderness.
6. **Malic acid** is found in apples and improves pain and tenderness.
7. **L-tryptophan** levels are often lower in fibromyalgia patients. S-hydroxy-L-tryptophan may help tender points, anxiety, pain, sleep, and fatigue after 90 days with a dosage of 100 mg, three times a day.

Exercise

Cardiovascular exercise has been found helpful to rehabilitate fibromyalgia sufferers. Patients are advised to perform active aerobic exercise three times a week for at least 20 minutes. The body's endorphins are thought to offer pain relief. Research showed that after 12 months of aerobic exercise, 55 percent of subjects with fibromyalgia, now met the criterion of not having fibromyalgia. Strength training is also important because it enhances growth hormone production. A review of 17 studies involving 724 fibromyalgia patients found aerobic exercise training had beneficial effects on physical capacity and alleviated symptoms of fibromyalgia.

Acupuncture

Acupuncture is the treatment of choice for dealing with myofascial pain disorders or trigger point pain. Treatment should be extended for several months for fibromyalgia patients. One acupuncture study found 46 percent of myofascial pain subjects had the longest relief of symptoms. In one controlled acupuncture study on 70 patients, 25 percent improved markedly, 50 percent had satisfactory relief, and 25 percent had no benefit for their fibromyalgia. Studies have shown electroacupuncture also to be effective. Acupuncture increases microcirculation blood flow over tender points in fibromyalgia patients, thus reducing pain.

Diet

A Finnish study found a strict low salt, uncooked vegan diet rich in lacto bacteria produced significant improvement in pain levels, joint stiffness, quality of sleep, and general health. Other studies confirm the benefits of a vegan diet for fibromyalgia.

Blood Type and Gluten

Research has found fibromyalgia patients with type O blood have a dramatic improvement in symptoms if they stick to a wheat free diet, gluten free.

Lectin is another possible dietary source that exacerbates fibromyalgia. It may facilitate the transportation of both dietary and gut pathogens to peripheral tissue resulting in fibromyalgia symptoms and rheumatoid arthritis.

Toxins

Controlled studies have found that fibromyalgia symptoms can drastically be relieved if certain exotoxins can be eliminated from the diet such as monosodium glutamine (MSG) and aspartame.

Homeopathy

A specific homeopathy remedy called *rhustox* has been effective in treating fibromyalgia. A controlled study on 30 patients found a significant reduction in tender points, pain, and sleep disturbances. A second study found it reduced pain in 52 percent of patients.

Hydrotherapy

Pool exercise studies have found fibromyalgia subjects significantly improved in physical function, grip strength, pain level, psychological distress, and quality of life.

Balneotherapy is one form of hydrotherapy. A study on 39 patients found it significantly reduced pain in fibromyalgia and the addition of valerian to the fresh water improved well being and sleep.

Magnet Therapy

Magnets produce energy in the form of magnetic fields and have long been used in healing and for treating pain. Two studies have confirmed magnets help with fibromyalgia pain.

Cannabinoid (Marijuana)

Marijuana can block nociceptive mechanisms in the central nervous system to reduce pain. Studies show it is effective with fibromyalgia.

Meditation

Meditation has been well studied with research showing regular meditation can profoundly affect the physical process and benefit overall health. Chronic pain and anxiety are helped by meditation, and it is particularly effective for fibromyalgia, especially when combined with mind-body techniques.

Low Energy Laser Therapy

Laser therapy is used for soft tissue injuries. By emitting a gentle energy, it can penetrate deep into the tissue without damage. The light stimulates cell repair, increases circulation, and relieves inflammation and pain. Many countries have approved low energy laser therapy for healing, but not yet in the United States. The treatment takes five minutes in a series of 15 visits. Laser therapy has been used effectively for fibromyalgia.

Guaifenesin

Guaifenesin is found in many cough syrups and decongestants. It supposedly gets rid of excess phosphates in cells of fibromyalgia patients. Some claim it will cure fibromyalgia, but no studies have confirmed its effectiveness.

Melatonin
Studies have found melatonin helps fibromyalgia patients sleep. A 1998 study found fibromyalgia women slept better after a nightly dose of 2 mg.

For a disorder that was not given a name until 1987, fibromyalgia has sure caused much suffering. Hopefully science can come up with a cure and provide relief. Thank goodness there are a number of alternatives that help fibromyalgia but one has to do homework to discover them and be diligent to find a solution for the pain and fatigue. Good luck!

Chapter Eight

Headaches

It Is In Your Head

Headaches are believed to be the number one complaint reported to primary care physicians. The two most common headaches are tension headaches and migraine headaches. It is estimated that lifetime tension headaches have been experienced by 88 percent of women and 69 percent of men. Nearly 18 percent of women have a history of migraine headaches compared to 6 percent of men. In the United Kingdom, two thirds of the population reported a headache in the previous month in one survey. One study conducted on 1,000 adults over 65 years of age found 22 percent had three or more headaches during the previous year. Chronic headaches are experienced by 2 to 3 percent of the population, with risk factors such as snoring, caffeine, stress, co-morbid pain, obesity, and overuse of medication. A third type of headache called cluster headache is more uncommon, with fewer than 1 percent suffering from them.

Migraine Headaches

Migraine headaches are characterized by symptoms that may include nausea, vomiting, sensitivity to light, sensitivity to sound, visual phenomena such as flashing lights or an aura. The headache is most often unilateral with moderate to severe intensity. Migraines are intermittent, but when they occur, patients need to curtail their work activities. Each episode lasts approximately 4 to 72 hours, with the average migraine lasting 6 hours. Migraine sufferers report an average of 19.6 lost workdays annually because of absenteeism and reduced productivity. Employer cost for each migraine patient is estimated to be more than $3,000 annually.

During a migraine episode both neurological and vascular changes occur. The classical migraine begins with a warning called an aura, with the headache arriving 30 minutes later. Migraines usually begin as a dull ache that eventually turns into a throbbing pain. A cortical spread of depressed electrical activity occurs, moving from the rear to the front of the head contributes to the migraine aura.

A migraine is caused by the narrowing of the blood vessels in the brain, with the narrowing occurring during the aura stage, which feels like a tingling or numbness. This constriction of blood vessels is followed by a rapid dilation of blood vessels in both the brain and scalp. The throbbing sensation comes from pressure on nerves by the dilated blood vessels. Physicians have identified 127 different factors that could trigger a migraine attack. Migraines can be triggered by stress, fatigue, low blood sugar, hormone changes, and environmental factors such as odors, bright lights, and smoking to name just a few. One should avoid the triggers which may not stop the migraine but may reduce the frequency by half. About 25 percent of people can eliminate their headaches by avoiding problem foods. These foods contain an amino acid tyramine, a chemical causing blood vessels to dilate or swell. Foods containing tyramine include cheese, alcohol, citrus fruit, nuts, and chocolate. Foods with sodium nitrate should be avoided, which is found in hot dogs, bacon, and salami, because it also causes blood vessels to swell. Monosodium glutamate (MSG), a flavor enhancement in Chinese food and meat tenderizer, should also be avoided. Migraines can also be triggered by low levels of magnesium, which has been found to be low in migraine patients. Foods that contain magnesium include nuts, whole grains, and spinach.

Some women get migraines before their period. To prevent this, some physicians recommend taking 50 to 100 mg of vitamin B6 and 400 IU of vitamin E. There is also a direct relationship between depression and migraines.

Alternative Therapies for Migraines

Instant Relief

For instant relief there are several techniques that may help. They include:

1. Be in a dark environment.
2. Think hot thoughts such as imagining your hands growing warmer. Then use your mind to direct the blood flow out of the head into the hands. Placing your hands in hot water will not affect the pain, only the imagination will.
3. Some women get relief by making love. An orgasm inhibits the progress of the migraine by stimulating the brain limbic system.

Biofeedback

Studies show headache improvement rates with biofeedback are similar to the drug propranodal, with 55 percent improvement in both. Placebo improvement was 12.2 percent and no treatment improvement was 1.1 percent. Results from biofeedback, relaxation training, and combined behavioral treatment were about the same. No advantage was found using hypnosis or other psychological techniques. All behavioral treatment should be considered to prevent migraines. A review of 35 studies found a 43 percent reduction in headache activity by biofeedback and relaxation.

Acupuncture

A systemic review of the literature found acupuncture can prevent migraines. One study of 179 migraine sufferers suggested that acupuncture significantly reduced the number of patients who develop a full migraine within 48 hours. Studies comparing TENS (transcutaneous electric nerve stimulation), low dose laser therapy, and acupuncture found acupuncture was the best for migraine prevention.

Diet

A study conducted on 88 children with severe, frequent

migraines, found 93 percent improved on a low allergy diet. The role of food in provoking migraines was established by a double-blind challenge in 40 of the children. Research of 43 adult migraine sufferers found 71 percent were provoked by food allergies but not by placebo. Some trigger foods may include chocolate, cheese, shellfish, and red wine.

A strong cup of coffee can ward off a migraine by constricting blood vessels in the brain. Caffeine also offsets the widening of blood vessels that occur during the migraine. Caffeine is listed on the labels of several pain killers including Excedrin and Anacin.

Herbal Medicine

1. **Butterbur** was used in a study on 60 migraine patients and compared to a placebo. After 12 weeks, 45 percent of patients taking the butterbur herb were helped compared to 15 percent of placebo patients.

2. **Feverfew** is a daisy-like herb that could be a solution to migraine headaches. The herb was used by ancient Romans to cure fever. Three studies have found feverfew to alleviate the frequency and pain of migraines by more than 50 percent. Scientists believe feverfew works because of its effect on serotonin.

3. **Shutianning granule** is a Chinese patented herbal medicine that has been found to be helpful for migraine headaches. Another Chinese study found a combination of soy, isoflavones, dong quai, and black cohosh to be effective against migraines.

4. **Lavender** is a plant native to southern Europe and Mediterranean area used for centuries in healing. Lavender has been found effective for migraines.

Spinal Manipulation

Three controlled studies found spinal manipulation to be effective for migraines.

Co-enzyme Q 10
A controlled study on 42 migraine sufferers found that co-enzyme Q 10 was effective in reducing the number of migraine headaches.

Yoga
A controlled study conducted over four months found yoga and standard meditation reduced migraine headaches as compared to standard meditation alone.

Leisure
People who develop migraine headaches tend to be hard driving, responsible people. One study found that headaches were reduced by one half for those who pursued leisure activities. Another study on 40 migraine patients found when they exercised, and spent time pursuing art, music, or reading, they were able to reduce the frequency of migraines by 50 percent. Three migraine groups were studied including a biofeedback group, a music group, and control group. The group who listened to music two times a week for forty minutes had fewer migraines. The music was a tool to relax the patients who then practiced visualization of being relaxed.

Tension Headaches
Tension headaches are the most common type of headache, with 69 percent of men and 88 percent of women experiencing them during their lifetime. One study found that 38 percent of the population suffered from a headache during the past year. The current theory is that the muscles in the face, the scalp, and the neck contract putting the squeeze on the blood supply to the brain, resulting in a tension headache. There are two kinds of tension headaches.

1. Episodic headaches are caused by stress, hostility, and anxiety accounting for between 75 to 80 percent of tension headaches.
2. Chronic headaches are caused by chronic anxiety or hidden depression, occurring in 2 to 3 percent of the

population. They are defined as headaches that occur 15 or more days per month for at least six months.

Tension headaches are described as a bilateral dull ache, a pressure sensation, or cap-like pain usually located in the forehead, neck, and shoulder region. Studies show that 60 percent of tension headache sufferers experience them one day per month or less, with 40 percent experiencing them twice a month. Less than 5 percent experience tension headaches for more than 180 days during the year. Typically they occur from two to seven days a week and can last from one hour to all day. Chronic tension headaches have been known to last more than one year. Among subjects with migraine headaches, 62 percent had an existing tension headache. Stress is definitely a factor in tension headaches. High amounts of anger are associated with migraines but not in chronic tension headaches.

Alternative Therapies for Tension Headaches

A. *Instant relief*

1. Take a short nap.
2. Take a deep breath and then yawn.
3. Clench your fists and breathe in deeply. Then hold your breath and then breathe out slowly and let the body go limp, like a rag doll. Then yawn.
4. Take a hike or a brief walk around the block. Walking may ease the pain by releasing the body's natural pain killers, endorphins.
5. Exercise will also release endorphins.
6. An electric massage will produce vibration. It is used with moderate pressure on a specific spot on the head. Vibrations may offer pain relief for several hours. For chronic pain, lengthen the treatment to 30 to 45 minutes twice a day.
7. Use your hairbrush to give your scalp a massage. Brushing improves blood circulation.

B. A review of many controlled studies found *spinal manipulation (chiropractic), therapeutic touch, electrotherapy, and TENS* were helpful for tension headaches.
C. *Acupuncture* was found to be beneficial in eleven controlled studies.
D. *Biofeedback and relaxation* studies found that both relaxation and biofeedback were superior to no treatment or placebo therapy. A review of 78 studies involving 2,866 patients found that in 29 studies involving biofeedback, 47 percent of the patients improved. The 38 relaxation studies found 36 percent improvement compared to the placebo showing 20 percent improvement.

Biofeedback strategies include:
1. Relaxing imagery where you imagine being in a quiet scene.
2. Repeat relaxing phrases over and over again.
3. The deep breathing technique has the subject repeating a relaxing phrase such as 'calm' when exhaling. Limit the pace of breathing to no more than 12 breaths a minute.
4. Be aware of tightness and tension in the body. Imagine what it would be like without tension in those muscles.
5. Nothingness involves the patient making their mind blank and thinking of nothing.
6. Mental games such as focusing on a color will help relax muscle tension.
7. Concentration on auditory feedback may help one relax.

E. *Exercise* has been found in many studies to be effective for headaches. One study found workplace exercise reduced headaches during a four week period. Regular exercise can prevent headaches. Walking, biking, or swimming, all increase blood circulation and provide tissue with more oxygen. Exercise causes the body to produce endorphins, the body's pain killing chemical.

F. *Herbal medicine* in controlled studies found *peppermint oil* was superior to a placebo but not different from analgesic drugs for relieving headache pain. *Tiger balm* was found to be better than a placebo at reducing headache intensity.

G. *Hypnotherapy* in the form of self-hypnosis was found to be effective on subjects who were easily hypnotized. There was significant reduction in headaches.

H. *Relaxation techniques* were found in controlled studies to have a positive effect on tension headaches. After four years, those who practiced relaxation were still being helped. Through relaxation therapy, the patient learns how to decrease the amount of tension in areas of the body. Using relaxation exercises when a headache is coming on can reduce the intensity. There are 14 muscle groups that can be relaxed. Relaxation therapy involves achieving a mental and physical state of tranquility in a brief period of time. One can apply these relaxation skills to their daily life.

I. *Cranial electrotherapy* involves applying a high frequency, low intensity current transcranially. It was found to be more effective than a placebo in relieving and reducing headaches.

J. *Noncontact therapeutic massage* was found to be more effective than a placebo in relieving headaches, with the effect lasting for four hours.

K. *Yoga therapy* was found to be effective against headaches in several studies.

L. *TENS (transcutaneous electric nerve stimulation)* involves rubber electrodes applied to the skin. Stimulation is done one to four times daily for 30 minutes to an hour. TENS can be done at home. Studies have shown TENS to be effective for tension headaches.

M. *Vinegar* also is an effective remedy for headaches. Add a dash of apple cider vinegar to water in a vaporizer and inhale the vapor for five minutes. Lie down in a quiet environment and the headaches should be relieved in 20 minutes.

N. *Acupressure* is effective for headaches as discovered by the Chinese in ancient times when they pressed certain points on the body and found headache pain would be relieved.

Technique One
Sit comfortably. You can find the two pain-relief points one-half inch below the base of the skull. Each is about one half inch out from the middle of the neck. Press into these sensitive areas with your thumbs for about a minute. Tilt your head back as you do so.

Technique Two
Locate a point in the webbing between the thumb and index finger where the muscle mounds. If you press your thumb and index finger together, the muscle bulges out. This is the mound. Find the point, then spread your thumb and finger apart, and press in toward the bone of the hand for one minute. Make sure you do this technique in both hands. These points will relieve pain in frontal headaches.

Technique Three
Acupressure on the foot will also relieve headaches. Take your shoes off. Place your index fingers on each foot between the big toe and second toe. Slide the fingers up two inches along the groove between the bones. Now press firmly in toward the bone that attaches to the second toe for one minute. You can also rub this point briskly for about 30 seconds.

Cluster Headaches

The third type of headache is a cluster headache, which is an intense headache around the eye orbit or above it lasting between 15 minutes to 3 hours. Cluster headache is named because the headache attack occurs in clusters, up to eight per day over a period of time, and then followed by an interval free of headache. Often the headache begins after falling asleep and also in the early morning. Many begin between 6 P.M. and 8 P.M. During a cluster headache, the pain builds gradually and relentlessly, then diminishes slowly. After the age of 20 is when they are first encountered.

Some researchers believe the cluster headache is related to dysfunction of the hypothalamus leading to stimulation of the trigeminal nerve causing the headache cluster. Others believe they may be due to blood vessel dilation, inflammation, or pressure on the nerve behind the eye, or perhaps a decrease of oxygen in the blood. Males suffer cluster headaches about six times more frequently than females. Studies have found that cluster headache sufferers tend to drink and smoke more frequently than the average person. Triggers that may set off a cluster headache include stress, sunlight, or nitrates in food. Because a cluster headache is vascular in origin and psycho-social stress is known to produce vascular headaches, one should try to avoid stressful situations.

For instant relief of cluster headaches, take a breath of pure oxygen which can be a pain stopper. Evidence has shown that oxygen levels in the blood drop just before onset of cluster headaches. One non-controlled study found in 90 percent of cases, patients who breathed pure oxygen could stop a cluster headache within 15 minutes.

Standard treatment for vascular headaches has been a combination of relaxation training and thermal biofeedback. Studies have shown that about half of the patients following this protocol of relaxation and thermal biofeedback reduced headache activity by 50 percent. Vascular headaches include both migraines and cluster headaches. Thermal biofeedback involves patients warming their hands with their mind and then directing the blood flow out of the head into the hands. Sensory biofeedback will help you learn the process.

A number of alternatives have been suggested, and you will have to experiment which alternative works best for you. Give it time and don't give up too quickly if the therapy does not work the first time.

Chapter Nine

Other Pain Disorders
From Neuropathy to Feminine Pain

We have discussed the major pain disorders that affect humanity. There are many other disorders that have limited information about the benefits of natural remedies. Some of these disorders will be discussed in this chapter. Because pain is all encompassing on how it functions, many of the alternatives discussed in other chapters may apply to various pain disorders even though the research has not been done on the specific disorder. Most natural remedies are safe.

Neuropathy

Neuropathy pain is defined as pain arising as a direct consequence of a lesion or disease that affects the nervous system, initiated by a primary lesion, dysfunction, or degeneration in the peripheral nervous system or central nervous system.

Neuropathy pain description has many different characteristics which include:

1. Feels like an electric shock, or like a shooting or stabbing pain.
2. Pain can be evoked by a light touch.
3. The pain sensation is increased in response to a normal painful stimulus.

4. A hot or burning pain.

5. A tingling sensation, numbness, prickling, or pins and needles.

6. Quite painful when exposed to the cold.

There are a number of causes that can initiate neuropathy pain including:

1. Diabetic neuropathy

2. Post herpetic neuralgia

3. Post surgical pain

4. Trigeminal neuralgia

5. Complex regional pain syndrome

6. Chemotherapy pain

7. Secondary to tumor infiltration

8. HIV related neuropathy

9. Central nerve dysfunction

10. Central post-stroke pain

11. Multiple sclerosis pain

Between 1 and 2 percent of the population suffers from neuropathy. There is no good standard for diagnosing neuropathy pain. Those who suffer from neuropathy pain report significant impairment of general health. The pain is associated with severely reduced functioning in all aspects of daily activities and life in general. About 30 percent of patients referred to pain clinics have neuropathy pain.

The World Health Organization estimates 180 million people in the world suffer from diabetes, with between 16 to 28 percent of diabetics having neuropathy. In Britain and the United States, between 6 to 8 percent of the adult population are likely to have a painful neuropathy condition. In diabetes, neuropathy pain is associated with impaired glucose tolerance or it may be due to poor circulation to the nerve. Neuropathy pain is found more in females after the age of 60, twice as prevalent in manual workers and farmers compared to managers, and it is greater in rural areas. The risk of neuropathy increases with Type 2 diabetes, aging, and duration. After the age of 60, peripheral neuropathy occurs in more than 50 percent of patients with Type 2 diabetes.

Post herpetic neuralgia is pain that persists for more than one month after the onset of herpes zoster. It occurs in 30 percent of patients following acute zoster herpes and lasts for one year in 16 percent of patients. In post herpetic neuralgia, there is a localized painful vesicular rash caused by varicella zoster virus, the chicken pox virus. The pain occurs after the rash heals. Prompt treatment with the antivirus drug acyclovis decreases the pain severity. Zoster vaccine reduces the incidence by 60 percent.

Trigeminal neuralgia is unilateral facial pain that is recurrent, brief, and stabbing. It seems to be associated with blood vessels being in contact with the nerve. Pain can be so severe that patients may be suicidal.

Drug Therapy

Neuropathy pain is recognized as one of the most difficult pain syndromes to treat. The pain does not respond well to conventional therapy such as NSAIDs.

Nonconventional painkillers tend to work best which include:

1. Antiepileptic drugs such as carbamazepine and gabapentin.
2. Antidepressants such as amytriptyline and saarto wiffen.
3. Tricyclic antidepressants work well for diabetic neuropathy.

Neuropathy pain is most likely to be reduced when patients are treated with antiepileptic drugs such as gabapentin or a tricyclic antidepressant, the first line of defense. Gabapentin does not restore normal sensation but decreases the annoying sensation that occurs in numb areas. It does reduce the reliance on opiate medication.

Other medications used for neuropathy include lidocaine, which reduces pain severity by about 30 percent. Low doses of long acting opiates are beneficial in patients who have failed other types of therapy. Studies show low doses of methadone or sustained release of oxycodone are also effective in reducing chronic neuropathy symptoms.

Alternative Therapies for Neuropathy

Jonothan Wright, M.D., in his book *Treasury of Natural Cures* has found a number of natural remedies to be effective in treating neuropathy.

1. **Magnetic energy** has been effective in relieving neuropathy pain. It is expensive.

2. **Primrose oil** has been found to be effective in significantly reducing diabetic neuropathy pain in a double blind study. If taken daily, the effects were seen 6 to 12 months later.

3. **Alphalipoic acid** taken both intravenously and orally (600 mg) for three weeks was found to relieve diabetic neuropathy if taken daily.

4. **Capsaicin** is a topical cream (0.075 percent capsaicin) that reduces diabetic neuropathy pain by one-half for 50 percent of patients using it according to one study.

5. Uncontrolled clinical evidence has found diabetic neuropathy relief was found from injections of **biotin, vitamin B12, and oral vitamin B6.** At the Tahoma Clinic of Dr. Wright, they effectively use a combination injection of 10 mg biotin, 1,000 mcg of vitamin B12, and 50 mg of vitamin B6 in treating neuropathy pain. Injections are given daily for six weeks and then tapered to every other day for another six days. The shots can be self-administered.

6. A **vitamin D** study on Type 2 diabetics found 100 percent of diabetic patients had low levels of 25 hydroxy vitamin D. All patients were given 2,000 IU of vitamin D daily, which seemed to be effective. Dr. Wright advises that it is always wise to work with an M.D., D.O., or N.D. who are skilled and knowledgeable in natural nutrition and natural medicine.

Other Pain Disorders 143

7. **Acupuncture** has been found to be effective for diabetic neuropathy as has electro-acupuncture.
8. **Amniotic Stem Cell Therapy** may be the medicine of the future. Stem cells are natural cells found in the body that are responsible for healing damaged joints, cartilage, and muscles. Early clinical evidence suggests it is effective for neuralgia. For more detail, refer to Chapter Six, the arthritis chapter.

Abdominal Pain

Persistent abdominal pain occurs in 7.7 percent of adults according to a British study, with 9.3 percent of women and 5.3 percent of men suffering from it. Abdominal pain is one of the most common complaints seen by primary care physicians, accounting for 5 percent of all pain complaints made to the general practitioner.

Irritable Bowel Syndrome

Irritable bowel syndrome (IBS) accounts for 40 percent of all abdominal complaints to physicians. One study conducted on 40,000 individuals found 11.5 percent suffered from IBS, with a ratio of 1.7 women to each man. Another study found 15 percent of the western population suffers from IBS. IBS is described as a combination of lower abdominal pain, changes in bowel habits, bloating, and rectal urgency. The discomfort is associated with the altered bowel habits. Numerous studies have shown IBS patients have increased psychological distress, with psychological treatment being successful in eliminating the symptoms of IBS for many patients. Methods include psychotherapy, hypnotherapy, and cognitive behavioral therapy.

Indigestion

Fruit sugar digests quickly and can form gas bubbles when combined with slow digesting foods like protein and starches. Those who have weak digestion should eat fruits with tea or coffee, or wait an hour before eating other foods.

The digestion center is also an emotional center. We digest foods, thoughts, and feelings, writes Dr. Hadady. Powerful emotions can reduce healthy bile flow, resulting in pain.

Ginger tea works well with indigestion. Other herbs and spices effective for digestion include cardamon, fennel seeds, and bay leaf.

Acid Reflux

For acid reflux relief drink 1/4 cup of aloe vera mixed with warm water or juice. Aloe is alkaline and soothes the digestive tissue and relaxes muscle tension.

Ulcers

Ulcers often hurt more after eating or as a result of being hungry. For ulcers, one should drink aloe vera to correct digestive upsets. Aloe heals wounds, burns, acid reflux, and spasms.

Digestive acids can be reduced by adding more green alkaline vegetables to the diet. Try adding some cooling spices such as cumin and coriander to reduce digestive acids. Cabbage and homemade pickled vegetables are good for ulcers.

Candida

To relieve and prevent symptoms of candida albicans, one should add a drop of Australian tea tree oil to a cup of warm water in a porcelain cup, not plastic. Drink this in warm water or coffee. Also use a drop of the tea tree oil on your toothpaste every day. Daily acidophilus and plain yogurt will help replenish digestive enzymes.

Allergy Factors

Abdominal pain may also be caused by food allergies, lactose intolerance, gluten sensitivity, and low fiber intake. Avoid allergenic foods and eat more fiber.

Psychological factors

Patients seeking treatment for chronic abdominal pain have a higher prevalence of psychological distress. A large study of individuals with abdominal pain identified psychological distress as an important predictor of new abdominal pain. Subjects without abdominal pain who had the highest level of psychological distress were three times more likely to develop abdominal pain within three months compared to those without psychological distress.

Childhood abuse has been associated with development of abdominal pain in adulthood, especially gastrointestinal disorders. A survey of 226 gastrointestinal disorder patients found physical or sexual abuse in about one third of the patients. Another study of 206 female gastrointestinal patients revealed sexual abuse in 53 percent and physical abuse in 33 percent compared to patients without abuse (37 percent sexual and 2 percent physical).

Recurrent abdominal pain is defined as chronic pain (greater than three months) with three or more episodes of abdominal pain severe enough to interfere with activities. The prevalence increases during childhood with a female predominance after adolescence. The condition is not associated with an identifiable pathology. One study of 107 children found 45 percent had irritable bowel syndrome. Another study revealed 36 percent of children with recurrent abdominal pain developed migraines compared with 14 percent without recurrent childhood abdominal pain. About 25 percent of those children with recurrent abdominal pain will continue to experience symptoms into adulthood.

A review of 100 pediatric cases of recurrent abdominal pain identified a significant role that stress and anxiety play, with aggravated nonspecific abdominal pain in 48 percent of cases. Such stresses may include family separation, moving, or death of a loved one.

Carpel Tunnel Syndrome

Carpel tunnel syndrome is a neuropathy caused by compression of the median nerve within the carpel tunnel of the wrist. Injury, trauma, or repetitive movement of the wrists can lead to the syndrome. Alternative therapies include:

1. **Homeopathy arnica** was tested in two controlled studies involving 99 subjects. It was found to significantly reduce pain compared to a placebo in one study but not in the other study.
2. **Yoga** was found to significantly improve carpel tunnel pain in a controlled study after eight weeks of treatment.
3. **Massage** relieved carpel tunnel symptoms in one controlled study.

4. **Acupuncture, chiropractic, and magnets** were found to be effective in controlled studies for carpel tunnel syndrome.
5. **Vitamin B6** was not found to be effective after 10 to 12 weeks, but after the twelfth week it provided significant improvement for movement and discomfort in carpel tunnel syndrome.
6. **Dit Da Jow** is used in Chinese medicine for relieving pain and injuries. It is often found in martial arts shops. Dit da Jow is a linament full of herbs that is rubbed into the skin to heal bruises, spasms, strains, inflammation, and carpel tunnel syndrome. According to the Chinese, the pain disappears quickly because of the unblocking of qi energy and movement of blood by the medicinal ingredients. The Chinese say "where there is pain, there is no flow."

Cancer Pain

Approximately 75 percent of all cancer is diagnosed in adults over the age of 60 years, and 30 percent is diagnosed in adults over 75 years. Pain is either due to the cancer or its treatment. Approximately 70 percent of cancer patients report pain. In advanced cancer between 80 to 100 percent of cancer patients have pain.

Alternative Cancer Pain Therapies

1. **Acupuncture** studies have found it can alleviate nausea and vomiting and radiation-induced xerstomia in men receiving hormone therapy for prostate cancer.
2. **Aroma therapy and massage** studies reveal that these two modalities have positive short term effects on the well being of cancer patients.
3. Studies found that regular **exercise** reduces the severity of cancer treatment-related symptoms such as fatigue, nausea, and pain.
4. **Gingko biloba** was tested in a controlled study of 48 cancer patients that had upper extremity lymphoedema

following breast cancer. It reduced the heaviness feeling and pain.
5. **Hypnotherapy** studies found hypnotherapy to be effective in controlling pain, nausea, and vomiting. A review of all type of clinical investigations found that hypnotherapy can alleviate cancer pain.
6. A **reflexology** study on 23 breast and lung cancer patients found it to reduce anxiety and pain.
7. One **relaxation** study on 56 cancer patients found **breathing exercises, muscle relaxation, and imagery** was superior to no interaction in controlling the pain of cancer patients. Another study involving 96 women with advanced breast cancer also received relaxation training and were compared to a control group without such training. The relaxation group experienced a better quality of life.
8. **Cannaboid supplements (marijuana)** was found in 9 controlled studies to be just as effective as codeine in controlling cancer pain.

Post Surgical Pain

In 1996 there were 31.5 million outpatient surgeries and 40 million inpatient surgeries in 2001. Estimates from epidemiological studies vary widely about post surgical pain, ranging from 10 to 30 percent of patients reporting some degree of persistent pain following one year after surgery. A review of chronic pain studies following breast cancer surgery reported a prevalence of pain in 13 to 69 percent after six months. One study on 5,000 surgical patients found 25 percent were referred to chronic pain treatment centers. Between 10 to 15 percent of modified radical mastectomy patients had chronic pain after one year of surgery. Studies revealed between 61 and 70 percent of thoracotomy and amputation surgery patients had chronic pain. About 60 percent of amputees report phantom limb pain two years after surgery. In hernia-surgical patients, between 8.1 to 19 percent reported pain for up to six years after surgery. Pain intensity immediately following surgery can predict the intensity and duration of future pain.

Foods and herbs can increase bleeding during surgery, and bruising following surgery. The American Society of Anesthesiologists suggest patients stop taking all dietary supplements and herbs two to three weeks before surgery. Herbs that complicate surgery include garlic, ginkgo, cloud ear mushrooms, panax ginseng, kava, St. John's wort, valerian, vitamin E, and alcohol.

Post operative pain continues to be poorly controlled with a large percentage of patients experiencing moderate to severe pain. Preoperative anxiety is a significant predictor of postoperative pain and analgesic consumption. Psychological intervention can reduce postoperative pain, and hypnosis has been shown to significantly reduce postoperative pain.

Female Pain

Premenstrual Syndrome (PMS)

PMS is one of the most common problems experienced by women, but ironically it is not known what causes PMS or how it can be fixed. Holistic physician Jonathan Wright, M.D., in his book *Treasury of Natural Cures* has written about a number of natural remedies that seem to be effective for PMS.

Dr. Wright has found that intravenous magnesium and vitamin B6 can lessen or even eliminate severe menstruation cramping as it is happening. However, he discovered taking these nutrients as supplements won't relieve cramps immediately, but may lesson their severity over several months.

A study involving 71 women who suffered from premenstrual dysphoria disorder were given either L-tryptophan or a placebo from the time of ovulation to the third day of menstruation. When compared to a placebo, L-tryptophan resulted in improvement of mood swings, tension, and irritability. Researchers believed the brain level of serotonin was increased. The study used 2 gm of tryptophan three times daily.

Dr. Wright does not think a high dosage of L-tryptophan is necessary. He recommends taking 1,500 mg of L-tryptophan daily twice a day between meals with a small amount of juice. He also recommends 50 to 100 mg of vitamin B6, 100 to 150 mg of magnesium, and for some women he recommends 2 gm of gamma linolenic acid (GLP) each day. He has found this combination eliminates a majority of PMS symptoms.

L-tryptophan is no longer available in natural food stores but only through compounding pharmacies. For referral to a physician that can help you, Dr. Wright recommends calling the American College for Advancement in Medicine at (800) 532-3688.

Dr. Wright uses vitamin A to treat heavy menstrual bleeding, suggesting 50,000 international units of vitamin A (not beta carotene) daily. He found the majority of women return to a normal bleeding pattern in one to two months. He recommends taking this dosage for 30 days, and then reduce it to 15,000 to 25,000 IU to prevent recurrence.

Dr. Letha Hadady, who is a doctor of acupuncture, writes in her book *Naturally Pain Free* about herbs for PMS. She cautions that long term use of anti-inflammatory herbs is not usually recommended. The herbs she recommend include:

1. **Andrographic** is a shrub found in China, India, and southeast Asia. This anti-inflammatory herb is used by traditional Chinese medicine to support healthy digestion, the cardiovascular system, and for urinary symptoms. It is also effective for diabetes, sleep disorders, fever, cancer, and has been found very effective for pounding menstrual cramps.

2. **Black cherry** is an iron rich anti-inflammatory herb effective for gout and severe joint pain. One tablespoon of black cherry concentrate added to a glass of water will help regulate the period.

3. **Goji berries** are known to protect the liver, improve circulation, and prevent cancer. It is helpful for female issues. In tea form it aids in sleep. Herbologists think it should be taken by everyone over the age of 40.

Herbal Combinations

1. **Xiau Yao Wan** is an herbal remedy used to reduce PMS, bloating, cramping, chest pain, depression, anxiety, and temper. It is used primarily as a digestive formula.

2. **Channel Flow** is a pain formula made by Health Concerns

that relieves cramps, joint pain, and muscle, abdominal, and gynecological pain. This herbal remedy includes corydalis, angelica root, and peony for nerve pain. Channel Flow includes cinnamon and tang kuei to enhance circulation, and myrrh and frankincense to help prevent and dissolve fibroids.

3. **Crampbark** is a time-honored native women's remedy for menstrual pain by warming and relieving spasms and enhancing circulation.

4. **Three Immortal** pills by Health Concerns is formulated to treat inflammation and menopausal symptoms. The herbal remedy helps with palpitations, vertigo, tinnitus, depression, insomnia, lower back aches, burning of palms and soles, bleeding gums, and lowered sex drive.

   It contains testosterone precursor herbs epimedium and morinda plus blood tonic tang kuei, eclipta, liguitrum, and lycium. The pill contains herbs to reduce hot flashes.

5. **Amla 25** is named for the East Indian berry amla and has great rejuvenating properties because of its high tannin content. Amla 25 in pill form decreases high blood pressure, liver pain, gallbladder pain, and pain located on the right side of the ribs. Considered a Tibetan Precious Pill, it is used in hepatitis, cirrhosis, hernia, Addison's disease, diabetes, and chronic fatigue. Amla 25 is effective for menstrual discomfort.

6. **Agar 35** is the most common traditional compound used for all types of anxiety, stress, and fatigue. It is effective for low and upper back pain due to excess irritation. Agar 35 supports the kidneys, liver, blood, and circulation. Take one or two pills daily. It is safe.

If your health food store does not carry some of these supplements, it might be wise to get on the internet to find where to purchase them. The internet is also a good source of information for natural remedies for your specific pain disorder.

Chapter Ten

Nutrition and Pain

A Cause and Cure

As we have discovered in chapter one, inflammation is associated with most types of pain and disease. Inflammation disorders affect millions, with over 50 million people suffering from some type of arthritis. Approximately 21 million suffer from osteoarthritis and 2 million from rheumatoid arthritis. Other inflammatory diseases include allergies and non-allergic rhinitis which affect 39 million people, cardiovascular disease affecting 60 million people in the United States, and asthma another 17 million.

Inflammation is also involved in many types of cancer as well as Alzheimer's disease. In other words, inflammation is at the core of most pain and most disease. The food we eat is very influential on the cause of inflammation. Today, the typical western diet contains more than 30 times the pro-inflammatory nutrients than a century ago. Science has been able to identify these foods as well as anti-inflammatory foods. Once inflammation is under control, the disease will improve and the pain will subside.

Dietary Fat and Inflammation

Diet is one of the primary factors involved in inflammation. It is fast foods, convenience foods, packaged foods, soft drinks, and unbalanced nutrients that promote inflammation. Over the past century, highly processed foods, which are pro-inflammatory foods, have largely replaced the anti-inflammatory fresh and natural foods. This has resulted in chronic inflammation. It is the wrong kind of dietary fats that cause the inflammation process. Fats are not inherently bad for health but it is the imbalance in the types of fats consumed.

Gary Null, a Ph.D. nutritionist, gives evidence in his book entitled *Reverse Arthritis and Pain Naturally* that inflammation is the common link in the vast majority of lifestyle diseases. Diets are no longer rich in anti-inflammatory nutrients. Environmental pollution, extreme stress, lack of regular exercise, poor sleep patterns, and overweight conditions all contribute to inflammatory conditions that cause disease and pain. If the inflammatory process becomes excessive or chronic, its regulatory feedback is unable to work successfully and severe damage can occur. This chronic inflammation can lead to osteoarthritis, rheumatoid arthritis, gout, diabetes, multiple sclerosis, heart disease, and cancer.

The food industry is largely responsible for our unhealthy diet. Refining, processing, and industrial manipulation of foods have created a diet high in carbohydrates, unbalanced fat intake, and a low intake of fruits and vegetables. As a result, the diet contains 20 to 30 times more pro-inflammatory fats than anti-inflammatory fats and far fewer anti-inflammatory vitamins and vegetables. Studies have shown between 9 to 32 percent of North Americans consume five daily servings of fruits and vegetables, meaning the majority of people do not consume an adequate dietary source of vitamins and other micro nutrients. A study published in the *Journal of the American Dietetic Association* found that two thirds of carbohydrates consumed by American adults came from bread, soft drinks, cakes, cookies, and ice cream. The refined carbohydrates raise blood sugar and increase the risk for diabetes. Research has found this high carbohydrate and high glycemic diet raises blood sugar, increases inflammation, and increases C Reactive Protein. This diet leads to obesity, heart disease, arthritis, and chronic pain.

Dr. Gary Null believes the major cause of inflammation is the diet and increased consumption of fats of all types. Since

1970, the consumption of saturated fats, polyunsaturated fat, and mono-saturated fat has increased 63 percent. Healthy fat is necessary in our diet for cell membranes and hormones. Healthy fat can be found in seeds and nuts. Most fats that we need can be made by the body except for two polyunsaturated fats called essential fatty acids. They are linoleic acid (omega 6 fatty acid) and alpha-linolenic acid (omega 3 fatty acid). Both omega 6 and omega 3 fatty acids play a role in the cell membrane. The ratio of omega 6 and omega 3 fatty acids in the diet should be 1:1 or at the most 4:1. Because of society's dietary change, the current ratio is 10-20:1.

The process of inflammation mediators originates with arachidonic acid which belongs to the omega 6 family. It is found in all animal-based diets such as red meat and dairy products. When arachidonic acid is metabolized, it is broken down into components which cause inflammation, constrict blood vessels, and increase blood's ability to clot. Omega 3 fatty acids do the opposite. They halt inflammation. Both omega 3 and omega 6 fatty acids are broken down by the same enzyme. If the ratio of omega 6 and omega 3 is higher than 4:1, the enzyme prefers to metabolize the good omega 3 over omega 6. In a diet high in meat and dairy products, omega 6 takes over and causes inflammation. An anti-inflammatory diet is high in omega 3 fatty acids, which are found in green leafy vegetables, flax seeds, grains, legumes, salmon, cold-water fish, and walnuts. Farmed fish have oils high in omega 6 fatty acids and are inflammatory.

Linoleic acid (omega 6 fatty acid) is essential for health but today's diet provides too much of it. One of the main reasons for the high incidence of inflammatory disorders is the use of vegetable cooking oils. The body converts linoleic acid into arachidonic acid. This in turn is converted to powerful inflammatory compounds such as prostaglandin E2. The conversion is strongly influenced by a group of proteins such as interleukin 6 and C Reactive Protein, which in turn unleashes a variety of pro-inflammatory compounds.

Alpha linolenic acid (omega 3 fatty acid) is the source of many anti-inflammatory agents in the body. Enzymes convert omega 3 fatty acids to EPA (eicosapentacnoic acid) and DHA (docosahexaenoic acid) which are anti-inflammatory.

GLA (gamma linoleic acid) increases the body's level of prostaglandin E 1, which in turn prevents the omega 6 fatty acid from getting out of control. Research has proven that supplements which contain EPA, DHA, and GLA have anti-inflammatory properties for conditions such as arthritis, asthma, allergies, and other conditions.

The quantity of trans-fatty acids has greatly increased in processed foods. The food industry began to hydrogenate omega 6 fatty acids, which increased the amount of trans-fatty acids. Scientists began to discover that trans-fatty acids were far more hazardous to health than saturated fats found in butter and fatty meats. The trans-fatty acids inhibited more of the enzyme needed by omega 3 fatty acids than omega 6 fatty acids thereby interfering with anti-inflammatory compounds. Studies have now shown that trans-fatty acids increase the risk of heart disease, diabetes, and other inflammation diseases.

Free Radicals

Another factor which increases inflammation is oxidative stress. From oxygen molecules, the body produces defensive factors that have the capacity to kill bacteria, viruses, and cancer. These defense factors include peroxides, oxygen ions, and free radicals called reactive oxygen species. If they remain active after the time they defeat the microbe invaders, they will begin to damage the body itself. These free radicals can damage protein, lipids (fat), DNA, and all components of the cell. This oxidative stress initiates an inflammatory response, and if chronic, can lead to arthritis.

The body's main defense against free radicals is the antioxidant glutathione. One needs to supplement the body to help make glutathione. Vegetables that best supply the nutrients to manufacture glutathione include broccoli, Brussels sprouts, cabbage, asparagus, cauliflower, garlic, onions, avocados, and asparagus. Walnuts are another good source.

Environmental toxins cause oxidative stress. For example, heavy metals such as mercury found in dental amalgams should be eliminated because mercury causes free radicals, and it is always leaching from the filling. Mercury from dental fillings can cause a multitude of health problems including mental health problems and brain dysfunction. Smoking, air pollution, and pesticides can all create free radicals. People with arthritis should eat organic foods and avoid foods with GMO, which include all products with corn. Organic corn does not have GMOs. Many people are allergic to corn, wheat, peanuts, and dairy products. These allergies trigger the inflammation response.

The American Diet

Our diet at some level is the cause of most health problems. It can cause inflammation; it can produce free radicals; and it causes people to be overweight and obese, which is associated with so many degenerative diseases such as arthritis, heart disease, cancer, and diabetes. Dr. Gary Null writes, "It is critical to obtain the majority of our nutrients from alkalinizing food sources such as raw vegetables and fruits." Studies have shown a relationship between higher meat consumption and a higher prevalence of arthritis in both men and women. All meat is a source of arachidonic acid, which plays a key role in beginning the inflammation process that can lead to pain, swelling, and joint damage.

Many studies have been conducted on Seventh Day Adventists who mostly are vegetarians and live a healthy lifestyle. They have a longer life expectancy than other U.S. citizens, and have significantly less morbidity and mortality from chronic disease as compared to the rest of the population. A long range study was conducted among Seventh Day Adventists who ate meat and those who did not. The study found the meat eaters suffered from significantly more arthritis. Even those who ate meat once a week suffered from more arthritis.

Meat eaters tend to be heavier than non-meat eaters. A meta analysis of 36 studies on women and 24 studies on men found that vegetarians had a significantly lower body weight for men (7.7 kg or 16.9 lbs) and for women (3.3 kg or 7.3 lbs). The Body Mass Index was two points higher in the meat eaters. Meat consumption can lead to weight gain, which can lead to arthritis.

Obesity has become an epidemic in the United States. Two-thirds of Americans are overweight and one third are obese. By 2030, it is estimated that 50 percent or more of Americans will be obese. Medical costs will increase from $48 billion to $60 billion over current costs resulting from obesity. Children are affected as well. About 21 to 25 percent of American children and adolescents are overweight, and approximately 16 to 18 percent are obese. One study reported by the *Journal of The American Medical Association* found a correlation between bisphenol-A (BPA), a chemical used in plastics and packaging, and childhood obesity. BPA coats metal cans and is found in water pipes and refrigerators. BPA mimics estrogen during critical periods of development and encodes the body for obesity in the future. The study found that children with the highest levels of BPA in the urine were twice as likely to be obese compared to those with the lowest levels. Another study found 6.6 percent of American adults were classified as morbidly obese. Obesity is both a cause and result of arthritis. People often don't exercise if they are obese and thus become more overweight. Obesity negatively influences arthritis because of the mechanical load on joints. It increases the release of pro-inflammatory cytokines that promote joint destruction. Obesity has been linked to depression and anxiety which also is linked to chronic pain.

Null believes that we are largely powerless to fight the influence of the food industry, which is supported by unethical legislation. There is relentless advertising of unhealthy food products to children and adults that results in Americans eating unhealthy foods that cause obesity. It has become a gold mine for the multinational corporations who manufacture these processed foods, and for the medical system assigned to treat those unhealthy results states Null.

The American diet contains too many refined carbohydrates, too much fat, sugar, salt and artificial ingredients. This diet is destroying American health and leading to heart disease, diabetes, cancer, arthritis, and Alzheimer's disease. Without a regular supply of vitamins and minerals, micronutrients, and phytochemicals found in plants, it is nearly impossible to be healthy. The cells in our body are starving for nutrients. The American diet is leading to free radical damage, premature aging, degenerative disease, infections, arthritis, cancer, and chronic pain, writes Gary Null.

Many processed foods are addictive, designed by the food industry to sell more junk food. Certain foods take over the brain, just like certain drugs. In other words, people can be addicted to highly processed foods. Dopamine is a neurotransmitter in the brain that causes a feeling of well-being. The body seeks those foods that raise the dopamine level. Low levels of dopamine receptors are found in obese people. They will eat more to satisfy that well-being they seek. Certain foods cause the brain to act in ways that resemble addiction to cocaine, nicotine, and alcohol. Once the high wears off, the withdrawal is so unpleasant that people eat more to feel better. The right combination of sugar, fat, and salt are found in the vast majority of processed foods. This combination tends to make food addictive as discovered by the food companies that make them. Luckily, the loss of dopamine receptors is not permanent. Moderate exercise increases dopamine as well as other mood neurotransmitters such as serotonin and endorphins. Besides reducing anxiety and stress, regular exercise improves self esteem, brain function, and mood. The brain does not age as fast with exercise. A 1995 study found a significantly higher mortality rate in rheumatoid arthritis patients who were inactive.

Nutrition Solutions to Inflammation

Because inflammation leads to chronic pain, Jack Challem, in his book *The Inflammation Syndrome,* lists 15 solutions to fight the inflammation syndrome.

1. One should eat a variety of fresh and whole foods. Processed foods sold in boxes, cans, jars, and bottles should be limited.

2. Eat more fish, especially cold-water fish because they contain the most biological active omega 3 fatty acids. Eat at least 2 to 3 servings of fish a week. Fish with the largest concentration of omega 3 fatty acids include mackerel, Pacific herring, lake trout, king salmon, and Atlantic salmon. Avoid breaded and deep fried fish. Fish eaters need to be aware of mercury in fish. Selenium binds mercury, so selenium supplements might be considered.

Vegetarians can increase their EPA and DHA by sprinkling flaxseed on salads and vegetables. Flaxseed contains large amounts of omega 3 fatty acids and also comes in supplements in capsule form.

3. Meat eaters should eat meat from free range animals or those which are grass fed. Game meat contains large amounts of omega 3 fatty acids. Animals fed corn and other grains have been found to contain very little omega 3 fatty acids but have substituted saturated fats.

4. Eat a lot of vegetables, and the more colorful the better. Vegetables and fruits are the best dietary source of antioxidants, which help counteract an overactive immune system The majority of antioxidants are a family of vitamin-like nutrients known as polyphenolic flavonoids. Over 5,000 flavonoids have been identified in plants. Quercetin is one type of anti-inflammatory flavonoid found in apples and onions. A small apple contains about 5.7 mg of vitamin C. It also has more than 500 mg of antioxidant polyphenols and flavonoids, which together equal about 1,500 mg of vitamin C.

   Vegetables and fruits are a good source of carotenoids, another family of powerful antioxidants. Of the 600 carotenoids discovered, several are important to humans, which include alpha-carotene, beta-carotene, lutein, and lycopine.

   One should eat at least five servings of vegetables and fruits a day. Try eating a variety.

5. Healthy spices and herbs should be used to flavor foods, such as basil, oregano, and garlic. Cayenne pepper contains a nutrient that blocks the transmission of pain between nerve cells.

6. When cooking, use olive oil as your primary cooking oil. Extra-virgin olive oil should be your primary cooking oil. It is rich in oleic acid (omega 9 fatty acid, an anti-inflammatory fatty acid). Olive oil also contains vitamin E and polyphenolic flavonoids.

Macadamia oil, grape seed oil, and canola oil are also good because they contain both omega 9 and omega 3 fatty acids.

7. Avoid conventional cooking oils because they have high omega 6 fatty acids and virtually no anti-inflammatory omega 3 and omega 9 fatty acids. Conventional cooking oils include corn, peanut, safflower, soy beans, sunflower, and cotton seed oils. Partially hydrogenated vegetable oils are the worst. These oils are found in salad dressings, non-dairy creamers, baking products, and many processed foods. Among the very worst are vegetable shortening and hard margarine.

8. Avoid foods and identify foods that you are allergic to. Often people become allergic to foods they most often eat. Food allergies often occur in those foods that are addictive. Nutritionist Melissa Diane Smith writes in her book *Going Against the Grain* about gluten sensitivity. She believes that half of Americans have gluten intolerance at some level. Gluten is found in wheat and can damage the gut, leading to other allergies. Many people are sensitive to the night shade vegetables such as tomatoes, potatoes, egg plant, and pepper, and this can be a problem to those with rheumatoid arthritis.

9. If possible, avoid sugars, or at least limit them. Refined sugar is an empty calorie providing calories but no vitamins, minerals, or protein. Diets high in sugar and highly refined carbohydrates elevate the pro-inflammatory C Reactive Protein. In a typical year, the average American consumes 53 gallons of soft drinks and consumes about 150 pounds of refined sugars.

10. Refined grains also provide empty calories and should be avoided. Wheat is the most common grain in the Western diet. Whole wheat contains more fiber and a few more vitamins and minerals. Wheat contains lectin, which is a family of proteins that interferes with absorption of vitamins and minerals. Loren Cordain, Ph.D., a professor at Colorado State University and author of *Paleo Diet* gives evidence that lectin may exacerbate the abnormal immune response of

rheumatoid arthritis. Brown rice is a carbohydrate that contains vitamins, minerals, protein, and no gluten.
11. Dairy products should be limited. Many people, especially Asians and Africans, lose their ability to digest milk following childhood. Cow's milk is a common allergen that contains saturated fat. Small amounts of cheese is all right for those without dairy allergies. Cheese does provide protein.
12. For snacks, eat nuts and seeds. Eating almonds, cashews, macadamia nuts, and pistachios may be good for your health. Nuts and seeds are relatively high in fat, and have a mixture of omega 6 and omega 3 fatty acids. Studies have shown that nut eaters have a reduced risk of heart disease. Both nuts and seeds are rich in magnesium which helps the heart.
13. When thirsty, drink water not soft drinks. Water should be your main drink. Teas are also good as they provide many antioxidant polyphenol flavonoids. Many studies have shown the health benefits of green tea, even for cancer.
14. Eat organically raised foods which are free of pesticides and GMOs. Many pesticides are estrogen mimics that simulate estrogen. Organic foods have higher vitamin and mineral content. Corn and grain fed to animals are not organic.
15. Reduce both carbohydrates and calories to lose weight. A 2002 study reported overweight was on the increase worldwide. The reason was thought to be the result of Americans exporting their unhealthy food habits to other nations. Fats cells that are located around the abdomen produce two powerful inflammatory substances, interleukin 6 and C Reactive Protein. Being overweight increases the risk of diabetes, heart disease, cancer, osteoarthritis, chronic pain and other inflammatory disorders.

Anti-Inflammation Supplements

For those suffering from chronic pain, it might be wise to supplement the anti-inflammation diet with anti-inflammation supplements. Many supplements have good science underlying their effectiveness. Before commencing on anti-inflammatory supplements, check with your health care practitioner, especially if you are taking blood thinners.

Omega 3 Fish Oils

Fish oils are rich in the anti-inflammatory nutrients EPA and DHA, with EPA being a major defender against inflammation. When consuming fish oils, the body does not have to undergo the many steps to convert omega 3 fatty acids to EPA. Over 2,000 studies on omega 3 fatty acids have been published in scientific journals. Studies show that omega 3 supplements and an omega 3 diet can significantly reduce inflammation promotion substances such as thromboxane B2, prostaglandin E2, interleukin 1, and C Reactive Protein. One study found that at the end of a year, 40 percent of patients taking fish oil capsules were able to lower their NSAIDs (non-steroid anti-inflammatory drugs), such as aspirin and ibuprofen. The risk of developing side effects from these NSAIDs were also reduced. Remember they kill over 16,000 people a year.

Fish oils also help rebuild articular cartilage in osteoarthritis. They reduce inflammation and inhibit the breakdown of cartilage. Fish oil deactivates the enzymes that break down cartilage.

A 25-year study conducted on nearly 13,000 men in seven countries found that elevated cholesterol levels were associated with heart disease only in locations where the intake of omega 3 and omega 9 fatty acids were low. A study of people eating the Mediterranean diet (high in fish, vegetables, and olive oil) found 50 to 70 percent of the people were less likely to suffer from a second heart attack during the four-year study. Fish oils are a natural blood thinner that help maintain a normal heart rhythm.

A 2004 study carried out at the University of Pittsburgh School of Medicine placed 120 arthritis patients on fish oil supplements containing omega 3 fatty acids for treatment of neck and low back pain that had resulted from disc disease and joint pain. The results were amazing with 59 percent experiencing decreased joint pain, and 68 percent were able to discontinue their NSAIDs.

University of California professor, Bruce Ames, Ph.D., discovered that fish oil can reduce cancer risks. It is known that at least 30 percent of cancer results from chronic inflammation and chronic infection. That figure might be much higher. Large amounts of omega 6 fatty acids in the form of corn and safflower oil promote the proliferation of breast and prostate cancer. A Swedish study found that fish eaters have one-half to one-third the risk of prostate cancer.

A controlled study on Crohn's disease patients as reported in the *New England Journal of Medicine* were given fish oil equivalent of 600 mg of EPA and 300 mg of DHA daily. After one year, 59 percent of patients taking fish oil were still in remission, twice that of the placebo group.

Flaxseed is a rich non-animal source of omega 3 fatty acids. Flaxseed comes in capsule form and can be purchased at the health food store.

Dosage: For inflammatory disorders, take one gram of omega 3 fish oil capsules daily. For arthritis, take three grams daily. For non-fish eaters, take five grams daily. Fish oils have a blood thinner effect so be careful if taking other blood thinners such as vitamin E, ginkgo, or coumadin.

Gamma-Linolenic Acid (GLA)

GLA is part of the omega 6 fatty acid family but behaves more like omega 3. It is found in seeds. Several studies have found it to benefit patients who suffer from rheumatoid arthritis pain. One study found it reduced joint pain by 36 percent, and the number of swollen joints were reduced by 28 percent.

Dosage: Take 1.4 grams to 2.8 gms of GLA daily. Side effects are rare.

Olive Oil

Olive oil is an omega 9 fatty acid abundant with oleic acid. Olive oil is very prevalent in the healthy Mediterranean diet. Diets high in olive oil have been found to reduce the likelihood of rheumatoid arthritis, with one study showing it lowered the risk by 61 percent.

Vitamin E

Vitamin E can significantly reduce a variety of biochemicals that produce inflammation, such as inteleukin 6 and C Reactive Protein. Studies suggest vitamin E is beneficial in Alzheimer's disease, arthritis, allergies, cancer and heart disease, all associated with inflammation. Vitamin E is an anti-coagulant that thins the blood and prevents abnormal blood clots. It is best if you take mixed tocopherol vitamin E.

An English study published in the *Lancet* involved 2,000 subjects with heart disease. Half were given either 400 IU or 800 IU of natural vitamin E. The other half received a placebo. After 18 months, the vitamin E group suffered 25 percent fewer non-fatal heart attacks than the placebo group. Four other large human trials involving vitamin E and heart disease found vitamin E was helpful against heart disease.

Natural vitamin E supplements can lower C Reactive Protein by 30 to 50 percent. A study involving 57 diabetics were given 800 IU of vitamin E for four weeks. C Reactive Proteins (CRP) were cut in half. CRP is a pro-inflammatory bio-chemical, and is a better indicator of predicting heart attacks than total cholesterol. Diabetes and insulin resistance are also associated with higher levels of CRP as is Alzheimer's disease, arthritis, and many types of cancer.

Studies have shown that vitamin E can reduce inflammation and pain in patients with rheumatoid arthritis as reported in the *Annals of Rheumatoid Arthritis* in 1997. A study involving British and German scientists treated 42 patients with 1,800 IU of vitamin E daily (900 IU, twice a day). On average, arthritis pain decreased by 50 percent of those taking vitamin E. Another 60 percent improved in the vitamin E group compared to 32 percent in the placebo group. Researchers believe vitamin E works by reducing nitric oxide, a free radical involved in pain sensation.

Dosage: 400 IU of vitamin E daily.

Glucosamine, Chondroitin, and Vitamin C

There have been many studies conducted on osteoarthritis patients finding glucosamine and chondroitin supplements were effective in relieving pain and restoring cartilage that protects the joints. Glucosamine stimulates the conversion of glycosaminoglycans to proteoglycans which gives resiliency. Chondroitin slows the breakdown of cartilage. Vitamin C is involved in some of the chemical reactions that form cartilage.

Cartilage breaks down throughout life and is replaced by new cartilage. Glucosamine and chondroitin help rebuild cartilage and have anti-inflammatory properties. Cartilage is composed of large amounts of collagen, and vitamin C plays an important role in synthesizing enzymes needed during the manufacture of collagen.

Dosages: People with osteoarthritis should take 1,200 to 1,500 mg of glucosamine and 1200 mg of chondroitin daily. Vitamin C dosage should be 500-1,000 mg daily.

Painless Diets

Nutritionist Gary Null, Ph.D., writes about various diets that have shown benefit in patients with rheumatoid arthritis. For patients who had been on the Mediterranean diet for six months, pain level and stiffness had decreased significantly in rheumatoid arthritis patients. The diet contains fish, vegetables, olive oil, and red wine.

An anti-inflammatory diet low in arachidonic acid, which is found in meat and dairy products, provides significant improvement in rheumatoid arthritis joint tenderness and stiffness compared to a control group. Inflammation factors such as leukotriene B4 and thromboxane were lower, especially when supplemented with fish oil.

In one study, a very low fat vegan diet provided improvement in rheumatoid arthritis patients' pain, tenderness, and stiffness. They lost weight and reported they were better able to function. All this happened within four weeks along with lower levels of C Reactive Protein.

A lacto-vegetarian diet for nine months also provides relief for rheumatoid arthritis pain, decreases swelling, and insures grip strength. The sedimentation rate, C Reactive Protein levels, white blood cell count, and health assessment scores all improved after one month and again after a year. The diet was an alkalizing anti-inflammatory vegan diet, with 75 percent raw food and 25 percent lightly cooked food. Pro-inflammatory foods such as refined carbohydrates, wheat, poultry, and shell fish were all eliminated. Subjects consumed no caffeine, alcohol, refined sugar, artificial sweeteners, or chemical additives such as preservatives and food coloring. No conventional table salt, deep fried or toasted foods, or night shade vegetables were consumed. Allowable foods in the diet included legumes, nuts, seeds, grains, brown rice, Essene bread, millet, and buckwheat. Beverages included herbal tea and non-dairy milk such as almond, rice, or oat milk. Filtered water was consumed as were fresh squeezed organic fruit and vegetable juices. Raw honey and natural fruit sweeteners were also allowed. For cooking, grape seed oil, sesame seed oil, and extra-virgin olive oil were used. Nine to twelve servings of fruits and vegetables were a big part of the diet. Anti-inflammatory fruits included red grapes, apples, citrus, papaya, berries, and pomegranate. Juicing was done on the fruits and vegetables. Spices and herbs allowed were cayenne, curcumin, cinnamon, thyme, and chile pepper. Protein smoothies were consumed for breakfast. The anti-inflammatory diet not only helps pain but also is good for preventing other degenerative diseases associated with the aging process.

In his book entitled *Arthritis RX*, Vijay Vad, M.D., professor of sports medicine at Weill Medical College of Cornell University, lists the most highly recommend foods for arthritis. Listed in alphabetical order, they include: almonds, apples, apricots, avocados, bananas, broccoli, cabbage, cantaloup, carrots, celery, kale, flaxseed oil, ginger, green tea, kiwi, olive oil, oranges, papaya, pineapples, potatoes, tofu, tomatoes, turmeric, and water.

Green tea is the least processed form of true tea containing the most powerful antioxidant polyphenols, especially epigallo catechin (EGCG) that expresses the interleukin-8 gene that is a key to arthritis inflammation. A study at Western Reserve University concluded that drinking four or more cups of green tea a day could help prevent rheumatoid arthritis or reduce symptoms.

For osteoarthritis patients, Norman Childers, Ph.D., found that by eliminating nightshade vegetables, arthritis symptoms could be eliminated. These vegetables include tomatoes, potatoes, pepper, eggplant, and tobacco.

Food allergies can contribute to rheumatoid arthritis. By identifying the allergenic food, Dr. Jonathan Wright, M.D., found that 40 to 50 percent of his patients had completely recovered from their symptoms. This is accomplished by the elimination diet to find what foods are allergens. One should start the diet by eating only foods that are less likely to cause allergies. Then add back to the diet foods normally eaten, and discover if you develop symptoms after they are reintroduced. Some food ingredients and additives are linked to increased pain. They include caffeine, alcohol, monosodium glutamate (MSG), and aspartamine. Caffeine is an addictive stimulant found in coffee, tea, chocolate, and cocoa. Alcohol is a blood vessel dilator that may initiate migraines or make existing headaches worse. On the other hand, for centuries alcohol has been used for acute pain. People sensitive to monosodium glutamate may experience headaches. Aspartame (NutraSweet) has been associated with headaches.

Many vitamins, minerals, and herbs have been found to protect the body against inflammation and pain. The next chapter will discuss this in more detail.

Chapter Eleven

Herbs and Nutrients for Pain

From A to Z

Most of today's medicines have their origins in plants. Indigenous people knew what plants helped to heal their health maladies. Aspirin, the most popular drug of all time was derived from the bark of the willow tree. There are a multitude of herbs and nutrients that are beneficial for pain. Most of the herbs mentioned in this chapter have been scientifically researched at some level, but some have not. Herbs usually have no side effects. However, some of these herbs can react with prescription drugs so it is always wise to consult with your physician before embarking on herbal therapy. Many of these pain relievers are anti-inflammatory. Some are anticoagulants and thin the blood. If one is taking a blood thinner, it is important to consult with your physician. For people who take garlic, ginger, gingko, ginseng, GLA, fish oil, chondroitin, bromelain, and vitamin E, they need to be reminded that these supplements can increase the effect of blood thinning drugs. For women it might be riskier during pregnancy and lactation with the limited amount of research on these natural remedies. The following is a brief summary of the many herbs and nutrients that have been beneficial for pain.

Aloe Vera

Aloe vera is a desert plant that has been used medicinally for millennia to treat wounds and gastrointestinal problems. The flesh of the aloe leaves when used fresh are prepared in a gel to treat scrapes and burns. Aloe reduces inflammation and promotes healing. The gel from the leaf's center can be made into a drink and used for arthritis, ulcers, and a laxative. Animal studies have found it to be effective, but no good arthritis studies have been conducted on humans. Drinking aloe juice reduces inflammation, pain, acid indigestion, menstrual cramps, and a variety of discomforts. It soothes sunburns and accelerates healing.

Nutritionist Dr. Gary Null in his book *Reverse Arthritis and Pain Naturally* states that aloe vera helps clean toxins from the body that may be causing arthritis. He suggests drinking two ounces of aloe vera juice twice daily on an empty stomach.

Arnica

Native to Europe, arnica is an herbaceous plant found in the mountain regions and deserts. Traditionally it has been used to relieve pain from bruised tissue, joints, muscles, arthritis, burns, ulcers, and excema. Arnica can raise blood pressure. Today, arnica is used in homeopathy where it is diluted. Several double blind studies suggest homeopathic arnica can relieve muscle soreness. If taken internally, arnica is toxic except in diluted homeopathic preparations. Homeopathists use it to treat joint disease because of its anti-inflammatory properties. Most pharmacies carry arnica cream for pain and bruising.

Agar 35

Agar 35 is considered the most common traditional compound for all types of anxiety, stress, and fatigue. The compound relieves both lower and upper back pain caused by excessive irritation. It supports the kidney, liver, blood, and overall circulation. Agar 35 has been used successfully for anxiety disorders, obsessive compulsive disorders, and post traumatic stress disorders. Take one or two pills daily. It is safe.

Amla 25

Amla 25 is named for the East Indian berry amla. Because of its high tannin content, it has great rejuvenating properties. Amla 25 is an herbal combination pill used to decrease high blood pressure, and it relieves pain in the liver and gall bladder.

Ashwaganda

Sometimes called Indian ginseng, ashwaganda is considered an Asian panacea. Commonly used in Ayurvedic medicine, it comes from a vine in the tomato family. It calms the mind and promotes restful sleep. Ashwaganda is often used for aches in the lower back, nerve pain, muscle fatigue, and it helps people resist stress.

Dosage: For chronic arthritis, use one half teaspoon of ashwaganda and vidari kanda powder found in health food stores.

Avocado/Soybean (ASU)

A mixture of oils from avocado and soybeans has been shown to relieve osteoarthritis pain. It is called ASU (Avocado/soybean unsaponifibles). A 1998 French study was conducted on 164 people with severe osteoarthritis of the knee and hip. The group taking ASU showed significantly less pain and disability compared to those taking the placebo. A similar study found those taking ASU for three months needed fewer NSAIDs to control pain than the placebo group.

Dosage: 300-600 mg daily. Minor risks for pregnant and lactating women.

Black Cherry

Black cherry relieves pain because it is anti-inflammatory. It is also rich in iron. Gout and severe joint pain are helped by black cherry.

Dosage: Mix one teaspoon of black cherry concentrate to a glass of water.

Boswellia (Frankincense)

Boswellia serrata is an Asian tree that yields oils, gum, and other products when its bark is peeled away. For centuries, the gum has been used in Indian Ayurveic medicine for arthritis and musculoskeletal pain. Animal studies have shown boswellia inhibits leukotriene synthesis which contributes to inflammation. Two studies found boswellia, when combined with the herbs ginger, turmeric, and ashwaganda, gave significant pain relief. The herb has a long tradition of use for arthritis in Asia. It is useful in chronic arthritis, ulcerative colitis, Crohn's disease, menstrual pain, tumors, cancer, and asthma. Frankincense was used in ancient Egypt for embalming mummies.

Dosage: Boswellia comes in tablets, drops, and a salve. The usual dosage is 150 mg tablets three times daily for two to three months.

Bromelain

Bromelain is a protein digesting enzyme found in pineapples, with anti-inflammatory properties used for sprains, strains, and rheumatoid arthritis. A 1981 arthritic rat study found bromelain reduced inflammation better than several drugs including aspirin.

A non-controlled study in 1964 of 29 people with moderate to severe arthritis combined bromelain to their steroid therapy. Swelling decreased and mobility increased in 18 subjects, no change in 5, and swelling increased in 2.

Bromelain has been shown to reduce inflammation and swelling in the back, especially around the discs. One large medical center injected bromelain directly into the discs to relieve symptoms of disc herniation and rupture. It is also taken orally for blood pressure.

Butterbur (Pestilence Wort)

Butterbur was used in the Middle Ages to combat the plague. A study involving 60 migraine patients compared butterbur to a placebo. For those taking butterbur, 45 percent were helped compared to 15 percent of the placebo group. The prepared medication is called Petadolex.

Dosage: Three capsules, twice a day.

Cannabis (Marijuana)

The medicinal effects of cannabis have been known for years. Before aspirin was developed, cannabis was used as the primary pain reliever. Traditionally it has been used for headaches, migraines, childbirth, gastrointestinal disorders, and other pain syndromes. A review of nine controlled studies of cancer patients found it was just as effective as codeine in controlling pain. Controlled studies found it improved pain in multiple sclerosis subjects, spinal cord injury, limb amputation, chronic pain and neuropathic pain. A double blind study of 58 patients with rheumatoid arthritis found improvement in pain and movement.

The active chemical in marijuana is THC (delta-9-tetrahydrolcannabinol). THC acts upon specific sites of the brain called cannabinoid receptors. It is available by doctor's prescription in at least 24 states.

Dosage: Oral - 5 to 15 drops of tincture,
1 to 3 drops of fluid extract.

Inhalation - 6.5 to 19.5 mg for smoking

Dronabinol is the prescription for cancer.

Contraindications: For women who are pregnant and lactating, patients with cardiovascular disease, and those who suffer from seizure disorders should consult with their physician.

Side effects: Long term use is associated with mental health problems such as memory loss, dizziness, fuzzy thinking, and possibly schizophrenia.

Capsaicin (Cayenne Red Pepper)

Cayenne pepper contains capsaicin which prompts the release of endorphins, the body's natural pain reliever. It is thought to block pain by interfering with substance P, a chemical responsible for transmitting pain signals.

Capsaicin is most often used as a cream applied directly to the skin. It gives relief for both osteoarthritis and rheumatoid arthritis. The relief is temporary and needs to be used regularly to get relief. Capsaicin cream can be purchased over the counter, and is recommended by the American College of Rheumatology. One study found it reduced diabetic neuropathy pain by 50 percent for half the patients taking it.

Cat's Claw

Cat's claw is a vine that grows wild in the Peruvian Amazon, with a long history for treating inflammation. A 1998 animal study found cat's claw to be both anti-inflammatory and an antioxidant preventing inflammation and other cell damage. Rat studies suggest it may protect the gastrointestinal system from damage by NSAIDs. Osteoarthritis studies show it is effective in relieving pain.

Physiologically it lowers the pro-inflammatory prostaglandin PGE2 and inhibits NF-Kappa B, which is a protein that turns on inflammation-causing genes.

Dosage: Effective dosage is between 250 mg to 1,000 mg daily. Some practitioners suggest taking 500 to 1,000 mg three times daily.

Cat's claw may increase the risk of bleeding if taken with other blood thinners.

Chamomile

Chamomile is an herb rich in antioxidants that acts on the nervous system like a tranquilizer and muscle relaxant. It comes in tea, capsules, or tablets, and is best taken at night to help insomnia caused by back pain. The mild flavored tea is helpful for menstrual cramps, stomach pain, indigestion, and fever.

Chondroitin Sulfate

Chondroitin sulfate occurs naturally in cartilage and is thought to draw fluid into the tissue to give cartilage its elasticity. It also slows the breakdown of cartilage by protecting it from destructive enzymes. For years, Europeans have been using chondroitin for osteoarthritis. Studies have found it to help stop joint degeneration, improve function, and ease pain. One controlled study for over three years looked at osteoarthritis of finger joints. The chondroitin group had a significant decrease in new erosion of finger joints compared to the control group. Chondroitin is a slow acting supplement that takes two or more months for the effect to manifest.

Dosage: Recommended dosage is 1,200 mg daily divided into two doses. There are no serious side effects.

Chorella

Chorella is a type of algae that reduces oxidation damage to DNA and reduces various forms of inflammation. Studies have shown it helps prevent arthritis as well as relieving symptoms.

Collagen

Type II collagen therapy is being studied to treat rheumatoid arthritis and juvenile rheumatoid arthritis. This type of collagen, derived from animal collagen, suppresses the auto-immune response associated with rheumatoid arthritis that attacks healthy joints. In both animal and human studies, type II collagen taken orally has reduced inflammation and pain with rheumatoid arthritis subjects. There have been no or few side effects. A double blind study at Harvard tested 60 people who took small doses of type II chicken collagen. After three months, there was significant improvement in swelling and tender joints compared to the placebo group. Four people had complete remission. A larger study involving 224 subjects had good results at the lowest dosage of 20 mcg per day.

Comfrey

Comfrey root has been used in European folk medicine for ages, and is known as "knitbone" because it accelerates healing of fractures. The root stimulates the healing process in muscles, tendons, ligaments, bones, and spinal discs. Studies show it is effective in reducing pain and improves mobility in arthritis patients. One study found comfrey reduced acute back pain.

Dosage: Comfrey comes in tea, capsules, or tablets taken two or three times daily. Ointments are made with 5-20 percent comfrey.

Caution: Women who are pregnant or lactating should not take comfrey. Comfrey can cause liver damage and should not be taken for more than six weeks a year.

Crampbark

Native women have used crampbark for ages to relieve menstrual pain. Crampbark has a warm sensation that relieves muscle spasms by enhancing circulation. It is incorporated into a pill that has other herbs and is named 'Three Immortal' by Health Concerns. The remedy is formulated to treat inflammation, menopausal symptoms, depression, low back pain, burning of the palms and soles of feet, and it improves sex drive.

Devil's Claw

Devil's claw is a folk remedy that comes from an African plant with bumpy hooks covering the fruit. The root contains harpagoside, which is anti-inflammatory. In Africa it is used for arthritis, and in Europe for rheumatoid arthritis. A 1998 controlled study on subjects with chronic low back pain found devil's claw relieved pain significantly better than the placebo. Many studies have demonstrated it to be effective in arthritis because of its analgesic properties. One study found it more effective than the drug diacerhein. Ten studies conducted between 1982 and 2000 found devil's claw helped rheumatoid arthritis subjects' pain and mobility.

Dosage: It comes in tea, tincture, and capsules. The recommended dosage is 100 mg daily. Devil's claw appears to be safe.

Dulcamara

Dulcamara is a homeopathy remedy recommended for joint pain, especially for pain that is worse during damp weather. One should avoid taking it with meats, beverages, and toothpaste.

DHEA (dehydro-epiandrosterone)

DHEA is a mild male hormone made naturally in the body used to make testosterone and estrogen. Studies have shown it to be effective in relieving lupus pain, inflammation, and fatigue when given in 200 mg dosages. Scientists think that the estrogen-testosterone balance is off in lupus women. Low levels of DHEA are found in rheumatoid arthritis patients. DHEA is important for regulating the immune system. Arthritis sufferers should be tested for low DHEA, and if low one can take DHEA supplements.

DMSO (Dimethyl Sulfoxide)

DMSO is a by-product of wood processing used in paint thinner and antifreeze. In other countries, DMSO has many medical uses including pain relief for arthritis by relieving joint and soft tissue inflammation plus softening collagen. It has the ability to transport drugs across the cell membrane. During the mid 1960s, studies were halted on DMSO because of lens damage in the eyes of animals. No problems were detected in human eyes. In some countries, DMSO is given internally.

In Russia and other countries, DMSO is used for osteoarthritis and rheumatoid arthritis. Research confirms it relieves arthritis pain and increases function. Veterinarians use it in the United States for musculoskeletal disorders. The FDA has given approval for a bladder condition called interstitial cystitis.

Fever Few

Fever few is a daisy-like herb found in Asia Minor that appears to be a solution for migraine headaches. In ancient times it was used by the Romans to cure fevers. A 1978 study found it beneficial for people with arthritis and migraines. Both the frequency and pain in migraines were alleviated. A British study on 60 migraine subjects found fever few subjects had 24 percent fewer headaches than the control. Five double blind studies have shown it prevented migraines and reduced their frequency. It has also been successful for treating aches and rheumatism.

Cautions: Don't use fever few if pregnant or lactating. It is a blood thinner so beware of bleeding, and never use fever few longer than four months.

Gin-Soaked Raisins

The Arthritis Foundation Guide to Alternative Therapies reports that gin-soaked raisins seem to be effective for arthritis. Both grapes and raisins contain anti-inflammatory compounds.

Ginger

Ginger comes from the root of a beautiful lily that is a staple in Asian cooking. Ginger is anti-inflammatory and a pain killer. Biologically it inhibits production of prostaglandins and leukotrines that cause pain and swelling. Ginger has a biochemical structure similar to aspirin. Most patients with osteoarthritis and rheumatoid arthritis find relief from pain and swelling. A number of studies have been conducted on ginger. A 2001 study published in *Arthritis and Rheumatism* journal found ginger as effective as conventional pain killers. The dosage was 255 mg twice a day. It significantly reduced symptoms of knee arthritis with few side effects. A 2003 double blind study found pain and swelling was reduced in knee arthritis.

Dosage: One to four grams of powdered extract can be taken as tea every day. It also is sold in capsule and tablet form.

Caution: Pregnant and lactating women should not take it. It is a blood thinner so beware of bleeding.

Glucosamine

Glucosamine, a major supplement for arthritis, is most often used in combination with chondroitin sulfate. It is a major building block in the water loving proteoglycans that is part of the process that binds water in the cartilage matrix and stimulates cells that produce chondroitin in joints that produce collagen and proteoglycans. Glucosamine helps the body repair damaged cartilage, as well as reduce pain and improve joint function. Glucosamine is a nonprescription supplement sold in four forms including glucosamine sulfate. In Europe it is regulated and sold as a drug.

An Italian double blind study on 80 arthritic subjects found it reduced symptoms by 73 percent compared to 41 percent of the placebo group. Twenty percent of the glucosamine subjects became symptom free compared to none of the 40 placebo subjects. Another study conducted by the University of Bangkok on 60 osteoarthritic patients compared pain scores on a scale of 1 to 10. After five weeks, the overall pain score was 1.14 for glucosamine subjects compared to 6.71 for the placebo group. A Portuguese study on 1,208 patients found 95 percent had a positive response with glucosamine. Relief still occurred 6 to 12 weeks after treatment stopped. No side effects were found in 86 percent of the subjects. Gastro-intestinal discomfort was the chief side effect but disappeared in one to three weeks. Another

Portuguese study compared glucosamine sulfate to ibuprofen for knee osteoarthritis. At the end of eight weeks, the glucosamine subjects had a pain score of 0.8 compared to 2.2 for ibuprofen.

Dosage: For subjects between 125 and 200 pounds, the dosage should be 1,500 mg glucosamine and 1,200 mg of chondroitin. Dosage should be adjusted to pain level. Vitamin C and magnesium increase the effectiveness of both glucosamine and chondroitin sulfate.

Grape Seed Extract

Grape seed extract is rich in proanthrocyanidine, a biochemical that is anti-inflammatory. Grapes also contain resveratrol, the compound that blocks the cox-2 gene from being activated. Some scientists believe that resveratrol may turn out to be better than aspirin in fighting disease associated with cox-2 such as arthritis. Resveratrol also protects against cancer and can be found in red wine.

Green Tea

Green tea is the least processed form of true tea, which contains the most antioxidant polyphenoids that express the interleukin 8 gene, the key to the arthritis inflammation response. Research at Western Reserve University concluded that drinking four or more cups of green tea daily could help prevent rheumatoid arthritis and reduce its symptoms. Other studies found it reduced rates of arthritis in animals. In Japan, green tea is accepted as a cancer prevention.

Guan Jie Yan Wan

This Chinese herbal remedy is good for joint inflammation. One major ingredient is erythrinae bark, effective for lower back pain and knee pain. The remedy also contains barley, ginger, cinnamon, which all reduce swelling. It comes in pill form.

Guafemesia

Some healthcare practitioners have been successful in curing fibromyalgia symptoms and rheumatoid arthritis symptoms with guafemesia. It is found in many cough syrups and decongestants. In fibromyalgia, it is thought to get rid of excess cellular phosphates. No studies have been done to confirm its effectiveness in either disease. Because it mobilizes uric acid from the body, it is thought to be effective with kidney stones.

Guggal

Guggal is an herb used in Ayurvedic medicine that can be purchased in American health food stores. Ayurvedic medicine believes that chronic pain may result from a variety of causes including toxins and inflammation of muscles and joints. Guggal is both a stimulant and detoxifier. For pain relief, it is often added to an Ayurvedic formula for arthritis and heart care. It improves circulation and relieves muscle and joint stiffness and pain.

Dosage: Take two 375 mg capsules, once or twice daily.

Horse Chestnut

The horse chestnut tree is native to southern Europe and today is found around the world. With its anti-inflammatory properties, it is used to treat pain and chronic venous insufficiency. Six of seven clinical studies found horse chestnut relieves leg pain.

Dosage: 100-150 mg daily in divided doses.

Contraindications: Pregnancy, lactation, and bleeding disorders. It does interact with aspirin and other anti-coagulants.

Lavender

Lavender is a plant native to southern Europe and the Mediterranean region used for centuries for medicinal purposes. It is rich in antioxidants that have been used for migraine headaches, neuralgia, bruises, burns, and other pain syndromes. Clinical studies have shown it to be effective in low back pain. Lavender aroma therapy is effective for neck pain. It is also good for anxiety and insomnia.

Dosage: Mix one to two spoons of dried lavender flowers in 150 ml of hot water. In aroma therapy, use two to four drops in two or three cups of boiling water.

Contraindications: Pregnant and lactating women should

avoid lavender. It can potentiate the effects of central nervous system depressants.

Mulberry Leaf Tea

Carbohydrates, such as bread, pasta, and potatoes, can be a serious pain trigger for many people. An enzyme in the mulberry leaf inhibits absorption of carbohydrates in the intestine. For centuries, Chinese herbalists have been using mulberry leaves as herbal medicine. For type II diabetes, it lowers blood sugar. Mulberry leaf tea also reduces chronic joint pain and rheumatism. It does this by reducing inflammation, reducing acid buildup, adds water to lubricate muscles and joints, and allows carbohydrates to pass through the body.

Melatonin

Melatonin is a natural hormone regulating the biological clock which controls the sleep/awake cycle and regulates sleep. Supposedly it slows aging, boosts the immune system, and improves sex. Sleep disorders are a symptom of fibromyalgia patients and melatonin has helped them sleep better. A 1998 study found fibromyalgia women sleep better after a nightly dose of 2 mg. Melatonin is not recommended for people with autoimmune diseases such as rheumatoid arthritis.

MSM (Methylsufonylmethane)

MSM has been promoted as the newest cure for arthritis without any scientific evidence. It is formed from the breakdown of DMSO and is found in fresh fruits, vegetables, milk, fish, and grains but is destroyed during food processing. MSM has the anti-inflammatory qualities of DMSO and is safe. Mice studies found it eased rheumatoid arthritis symptoms but no human studies have been conducted.

Nettles

Stinging nettles are an irritating weed but have been found to ease painful joints and rheumatoid flare ups. Most often nettles are taken in the form of an extract or by eating the cooked leaves. Nettles contain boron, found to be helpful in osteoarthritis and rheumatoid arthritis, and other anti-inflammatory chemicals. A German study conducted on 40 osteoarthritis subjects who were given 50 mg of nettles and one-fourth dose of diclofenal (an NSAID). Pain and stiffness improved, and protein serum levels improved by 70 percent. Studies have shown it to be effective in arthritis of the fingers, prostate hyperplasia, and chronic arthritis.

Peppermint

Peppermint contains salicylates which relieve pain. Aspirin is a salicylate. One controlled study found peppermint superior to a placebo in relieving pain but not different from analgesic drugs. Peppermint is used as a local anaesthetic for headaches and also relieves itching. Neuralgia is helped by peppermint as are tension headaches, irritable bowel syndrome, and myalgia.

Dosage: Peppermint Leaf – 3 to 6 gm daily: Dry Extract – 0.8 to 1.8 gm daily

Contraindications: Women who are pregnant and lactating, and children under 12.

Phytodolor Tincture

Phytodolor is a preparation of herbs found to reduce pain in six double blind studies. It consists of European ash bark, leaves or bark of European aspen, and golden rod. Phytodolor is anti-inflammatory. It relieves spasm, musculoskeletal pain, rheumatoid disorders, low back pain, neuralgia, and osteoarthritis.

Primrose

Evening primrose is a plant native to North America used to treat a variety of conditions by its anti-inflammatory properties. Today primrose is used for menopausal women, gastrointestinal disorders, rheumatoid disorders, PMS, dementia, and cardiovascular conditions. Scientific studies have shown it to be effective with rheumatoid arthritis and diabetic neuropathy.

Dosage: 3 to 8 gm daily in divided doses.

Contraindications: Pregnancy, lactation, epilepsy, and mania.

Side Effects: Primrose is considered generally safe.
Occasionally there will be gastrointestinal symptoms and headaches. It can interact with anti-inflammatory drugs.

Resinall E and Resinall K

Resinall is an herb used for excess bleeding and pain during and following surgery. It reduces swelling, helps arthritic pain, promotes tissue regeneration, and activates circulation. Topically, resinall is used for fungal infections.

Red Clover

Red clover is native to most of Europe and was brought to the United States. Used by both Chinese and Russian folk healers, red clover is used in cancer, menopausal conditions, and mastalgia. Eleven controlled studies found red clover reduced hot flashes.

S-adenosyl-L-methionine (SAM-e)

SAM-e is a naturally occurring molecule present in all parts of the body. People with low vitamin B12 and folate deficiencies may have low SAM-e levels. It contributes to activation and metabolism of hormones, neurotransmitters, and proteins. SAM-e has both analgesic and anti-inflammatory effects, and has the ability to stimulate cartilage growth and increase dopamine and noradrenaline. Conditions frequently treated include osteoarthritis, fibromyalgia, musculoskeletal pain, migraines, depression, and Alzheimer's disease. Studies have found it to be very effective in improving functions of osteoarthritis patients and as effective in reducing pain as NSAIDs. SAM-e was found to be as effective as Celebrex in reducing osteoarthritis pain but has a slower onset.

Dosage: 400 to 1,600 mg daily. There are few risks but SAM-e can interact with serotonin syndromes.

Salicylates

Salicylates block vitamin K which increases blood coagulation. In other words salicylates are blood thinners that reduce pain. Aspirin is a salicylate. There are a number of herbs and spices high in salicylates including curry powder, cayenne pepper, ginger, thyme, cinnamon, oregano, turmeric, licorice, and peppermint. Some fruits that are high in salicylates include raisins, prunes, cherries, cranberries, blueberries, grapes, strawberries, tangerines, and oranges. Other foods and drinks high in salicylates include honey, peppermint, vinegar, wine and cider.

Shark Cartilage

Shark cartilage is derived from hammerhead and dog fish sharks. Sharks never get cancer so shark cartilage is believed to be anti-cancerous. It is used in management of cancer pain and arthritis.

Dosage: 500 to 4,500 mg in divided doses. Be cautious with liver disease and don't use if pregnant or lactating.

Shilajit

Shilajit has been used for thousands of years in India, China, Tibet, and Russia, with some claiming it can prevent and cure every discomfort and disease known to man. Shilajit is a mineral pitch with bitumen and fulvic acid, which has amino acids and condensed minerals gathered from drips seeping from cracked rocks in the Himalayas during hot weather. Ayurvedic medicine finds Shilajit improves libido, stabilizes blood sugar, improves immunity, heals injuries, knits broken bones, and relieves back pain.

St. John's Wort

St. John's Wort is a small yellow wild flower that grows in Europe and the United States. It is well known for its ability to help depression because of hypericin and hyperforin that raise serotonin levels. St. John's wort is effective in chronic pain and the depression that accompanies it, and is available in tea, capsules, and tablets.

Dosage: 300 mg three times daily. It does interact with many drugs.

Thunder God Vine

In China, thunder god vine is used in many forms to treat autoimmune diseases. Animal studies have shown it to interfere with the production of biochemicals responsible for the immune response and inflammation. One study found small amounts of thunder god vine can inhibit the release of pain biochemicals.

Tiger Balm

Tiger balm is a supplement effective for relieving back pain by improving blood flow, which provides heat to soothe pain. Tiger balm is very effective for pain when applied at night before sleep, and is also effective for pain from temporal mandibular disorders. One study found tiger balm to be more effective than a placebo for reducing headache intensity.

Triphala

Triphala is an herbal pill made of dried powder from three medicinal fruits. Ayurvedic medicine uses it because of its anti-inflammatory properties. Triphala is very effective in treating rheumatic aches, pancreatic cancer, and obesity. It improves heart conditions, diabetes, vision, digestion, and nerve pain.

Dosage: Take one or two pills with meals for inflammation pain, PMS, and digestive problems.

Turmeric

Turmeric is a root related to ginger, commonly used in Ayurvedic medicine in India. Turmeric is useful in treating inflammation, clogged arteries, bruises, bursitis, and numerous painful conditions. In Traditional Chinese Medicine, turmeric is used to treat arthritis pain. Curcumin is the active ingredient. Animal studies found turmeric to inhibit certain prostaglandins. Several controlled studies found Turmeric relieved pain and inflammation in rheumatoid arthritis and osteoarthritis.

Dosage: 400 mg of turmeric, three times daily.

White Flower

White flower is a Chinese analgesic liquid recommended for muscle and joint pain, headaches, back pain, neuralgia, arthritis pain, spasm pain, and bruises. The White Flower remedy contains oils from menthol, camphor, peppermint, and lavender.

Willow Bark

Willow bark contains salicin, the active ingredient in aspirin. Being both anti-inflammatory and a pain reliever, willow bark comes in capsules, tablets, and tea. The bark was first mentioned in 700 BCE for its pain relieving ability. Today willow bark is used for rheumatoid arthritis, chronic pain, headaches, and even the common cold.

Dosage: Prepared medications include:
Assalix – 2 to 3 times daily
Assplant pills – 1 to 2 pills after meals

Yucca

Yucca comes from the yucca plant of western North America. Used as an herbal medicine that comes in capsule form, yucca reduces joint pain and swelling. Saponin is the active healing ingredient that makes the joint juicy. Yucca soothes, moistens, and cools painful knees.

Dosage: Two capsules daily equaling 980 mg.

Yunnan Paiyao

Yunnan paiyao is a Chinese herb good for bee stings, muscle aches, rheumatoid arthritis, backaches, and minor joint aches. It stops hemorrhaging and normalizes blood flow.

Valerian Root

Valerian is an excellent tranquilizer and muscle relaxant without side effects. If taken before bedtime, it promotes restful sleep. Valerian is a natural pain reliever and muscle relaxant. Fibromyalgia patients benefit from valerian's sleep properties.

SUPPLEMENTS THAT RELIEVE PAIN

Nutritionist Gary Null, Ph.D., recommends a number of supplements to help reduce pain. Antioxidant vitamins are at the top of his list. These vitamins target inflammation that can lead to chronic disease and pain.

For arthritis, Null suggests the best way to take supplements is to divide them into three separate batches. Begin by selecting six supplements and take them for three months. After three months, add in the next batch of six, and after another three months add in the remaining five supplements. It is preferable to start at lower doses and work up to higher doses. The recommended supplements include:

1. **Antioxidants**
   A. *Vitamin C*

   Vitamin C is an antioxidant good for inflammation and pain. Start at 500 mg a day of vitamin C and work up to 1,000 mg after one month if no symptoms. Not every one has the same tolerance. Null suggests working up to 3,000 mg. A Framingham study found high intakes of vitamin C decreased the risk of osteoarthritis by threefold. Usual dosage was 500-1,000 mg as recommended by the Arthritis Foundation.

   B. *Vitamin D*

   The Framingham study also found individuals who consumed low amounts of vitamin D had progression of osteoarthritis three times higher. Vitamin D is found in dairy products and is also synthesized in the body, particularly in the skin in response to sunlight. Usual dosage is 400-800 IU daily, but many health care practitioners suggest 2000 IU a day. Low vitamin D is now being associated with Alzheimer's disease.

   C. *Vitamin E*

   Vitamin E has been shown to help reduce the risk of heart disease. Several studies have shown vitamin E to relieve pain better than a placebo, while another study found it was better than an NSAID for relieving pain. The recommended dosage is 400 - 600 IU.

   D. *Vitamin A*

   Dr. Null recommends 50,000 IU of vitamin A. Beta carotene should also be taken to help prevent and reduce arthritis.

2. **Gamma Linolenic Acid (GLA)**
   GLA is high in prostaglandins that reduce inflammation and pain. It is found in evening primrose and black currant oils. Take 240 mg of GLA daily.

3. **Glucosamine**
   Glucosamine repairs cartilage and tissue damage. It is a safe supplement. Take 1,500-2,000 mg daily.

4. **Grape Seed Extract**
   Grape seeds contain pycnogenol, an antioxidant that strengthens collagen. Another antioxidant, proanthocynidines, is found in the seed. Take 100 mg each day.

5. **Niacinamide**
   Niacinamide is a form of vitamin B3. Take 150-250 mg before mealtime, three or four times a day. Often there is a gradual reduction of symptoms and improved range of motion. Don't confuse with niacin.

6. **Omega 3 Fatty Acids**
   Omega 3 fatty acid is anti-inflammatory containing both EPA and DHA. Good food sources are fish oil, walnut oil, flaxseed oil, chia seeds, salmon, and sardines. Omega 3 reduces arthritic pain. Take 2000 mg daily.

7. **Vitamin B Complex**
   Vitamin B complex helps regulate the nervous system and enhances the utilization of other nutrients. Take 15-50 mg of vitamin B1, 100 mg of vitamin B5, and 50 mg of vitamin B6.

   Folic acid is needed for cells to reproduce and is needed to maintain healthy cartilage. Adequate folic acid levels are important for people with rheumatoid arthritis who take methotrexate.

   Bioflavonoids are found in all plants and are essential for healthy capillary walls and for metabolism of vitamin C. There are 4,000 various types of bioflavonoids, which are antioxidants that reinforce collagen, The best sources are green tea, berries, onions, citrus foods, fresh fruit, and vegetables.

8. **Bromelain**
   Bromelain is an enzyme derived from pineapples that reduces pain and improves mobility. The dose depends on severity of knee pain.
9. **Decursinoc**
   Decursinoc is in a class called courmarins, which is anti-inflammatory and reduces pain through its anti-oxidant properties. The daily dose is 200 mg.
10. **Methylsulfonylmethane (MSM)**
    MSM is a natural sulfur found in the body that relieves joint pain and reduces inflammation. Take 500 mg daily.
11. **Probiotics**
    Probiotics are beneficial bacteria necessary for digestion and immunity. Each day take at least 5 billion colony forming units (CFU) which contain multiple strains.
12. **Quercetin**
    Quercetin is a naturally occurring flavonoid found in apples and onions. It is an anti-oxidant that magnifies the effect of vitamin C.
13. **S-adenosyl-L-methionine (SAM-e)**
    SAM-e helps restore white blood cell activity in joint fluid and reverses glutathione depletion, thereby protecting and rebuilding cartilage. Take 400 mg daily.
14. **Superoxide Dismutase (SOD)**
    SOD is a powerful antioxidant. Dr. Null suggests taking it with vitamin E. Take 2,000 mg with water on an empty stomach about one-half hour before meals. It often relieves arthritis.
15. **Vitamin K**
    Vitamin K is a potent anti-inflammatory vitamin that prevents and treats arthritis. Take 2 mg daily.

Minerals

A number of minerals help relieve arthritis pain. Dr. Null suggests talking to your physician or dietician about dosage because of variables of age, weight, and sex. Minerals which are helpful for healthy bones include calcium, phosphorous, boron, copper, and magnesium. Those essential for a healthy immune system include selenium and zinc. Null states that the daily intake should include all the minerals. Multiple vitamins contain many of them.

1. **Copper**
Copper is an essential trace mineral that helps in bone growth and helps bone loss. Being anti-inflammatory, copper boosts the activities of NSAID drugs without risking ulcers

    Folklore believes that wearing copper bracelets can relieve rheumatoid arthritis pain. Several controlled studies have confirmed this. A review of studies involving 1,500 patients between 1940 and 1971 found copper complexes helped relieve pain in patients with rheumatoid arthritis, ankylosing spondylitis, gout, and Reuters syndrome. The copper complex was given intravenously. Some side effects were nausea, vomiting, anemia, and diarrhea. Chocolate and nuts have high copper as do seeds and dried beans. The usual dosage is 1 mg to 3 mg daily of copper chelate. Multivitamins usually have copper doses of 2 mg.

2. **Magnesium**
Magnesium supplements often improve pain and fatigue. This mineral is found in nuts, grains, and whole foods. Studies have found it relieves fibromyalgia symptoms. Magnesium can interact with blood pressure medication and high doses can be toxic. If kidney problems, avoid. One side effect might be diarrhea.

3. **Selenium**
Selenium protects cells from oxidative damage. Often it is low in people with rheumatoid arthritis and other inflammatory conditions. A double blind study in Germany on rheumatoid arthritis patients found selenium supplements reduced joint tenderness, swelling, and morning stiffness at the end of six months. Dosage is 50 - 200 mcg daily. It is toxic at 900 mcg.

4. **Boron**
   Boron is a trace mineral that helps the body use calcium and magnesium. Studies have shown that boron can ease the symptoms of osteoarthritis, rheumatoid arthritis, and osteoporosis. Animal studies have shown boron to reduce rheumatoid arthritis effects and double the natural killer cell concentration that fights cancer. A double blind study found subjects who took six mg/day of boron had less leg pain, joint swelling, and better function than a placebo group. Boron is plentiful in many fruits, vegetables, dried beans, beer, wine, and cider.

5. **Zinc Sulfate**
   Zinc sulfate is often used to prevent colds. Studies have shown rheumatoid arthritis patients have low levels of zinc. A double blind study found zinc sulfate improved joint swelling, morning stiffness, walking time, and overall impression of helping the disease. A safe dosage is less than 50 mg daily.

Nutrition, herbs, and supplements are a proven method to reduce pain naturally with few side effects. It is always wise to consult with your health care practitioner before embarking on such a program.

Chapter Twelve

Natural Therapies for Pain

A Synopsis

We have discussed in detail many natural therapies that seem to be effective for pain relief including nutrition, herbs, vitamins, exercise, the mind, relaxation, cognitive behavior, and many more. Most were backed by good science. In this chapter we will discuss other natural pain remedies, perhaps not as thoroughly researched but still with good scientific evidence showing they are effective. The exception is acupuncture, which has many scientific studies confirming its effectiveness against pain.

Acupuncture

For more than 2,500 years acupuncture has been a reliable healing modality of Asian medicine to maintain health and treat disease. In Europe, it is practiced by more than 40,000 physicians in Germany. In the United States acupuncture has been widely accepted since 1993 after funding by the National Center for Complementary and Alternative Medicine under the National Institute for Health in Washington, D.C. Acupuncture treatment is offered in more than 80 percent of all pain therapy clinics. Studies have shown that acupuncture is highly successful in chronic pain patients.

The underlying concept of acupuncture assumes that by introducing needles into designated body areas, disease and pain can be positively influenced. It is believed that needles can regulate the flow of qi, the life force energy in the acupuncture meridians; expelling pathogenic factors; removing stagnation; and treating disharmonies of the inner organs. In other words, acupuncture corrects the flow of qi to promote optimal health. This is how the East explains why acupuncture works. The scientific West has a different explanation. They assert acupuncture is a repetitive stimulus that activates pain inhibiting mechanisms on nerves and hormone levels using local and systemic points of attack. If the West can explain it by traditional science, they are more likely to use it.

Studies have shown that acupuncture has an anti-inflammatory effect on tissues. There is a peripheral release of endorphins, the pain killing opioid hormone that may play a role in pain relief and anti-inflammation. Research has shown that endorphins are raised in the blood after acupuncture therapy. Acupuncture is known to be effective with myofascial pain, characterized by painful regions in muscles called trigger points. Certain acupoints correspond to these myofascial trigger points. A non-painful acupuncture procedure can also inhibit effects on nerves in the spinal cord.

Electro-acupuncture uses an electric charge applied to the needle. Release of various endorphin subclasses depend on the frequency of the electric needle stimulation. Low frequency electro-acupuncture leads to the release of beta-endorphins and encephalins in the brain, while high frequency releases dynorphia in the spinal cord. Acute pain should be treated at 20-100 Hz and chronic pain at 2-7 Hz.

Research has shown that acupuncture can modulate activities of the brain such as the cerebellum and sensory motor cortex. It also activates the hypothalamus, which represents the interface between nerves and the endocrine system. Animal studies found that acupuncture releases oxytocin, which has pain relieving effects and also increases serotonin levels which can relieve pain. This may explain why migraine sufferers are helped by acupuncture.

In a clinical setting of chronic pain patients, the therapeutic effect of acupuncture appears only after several sessions. Acupuncture treatment most often involves repetitive treatments. One thing that Western medicine can't explain is the long term effect of acupuncture. Perhaps they might need to look at the open qi energy channels.

A multitude of pain syndromes have been scientifically proven to be helped by acupuncture including arthritic pain, fibromyalgia, primary headaches, migraines, low back pain, chronic back pain, chronic neck pain, shoulder pain, Raynauds syndrome, cancer related pain, visceral pain of the organs, post operative nausea, chemotherapy nausea, dental pain, knee osteoarthritis pain, trigeminal neuralgia, neuropathy pain, and irritable bowel syndrome. Acupuncture in acute conditions such as a muscle spasm or backache respond within a few sessions, but chronic pain conditions associated with arthritis may take one or two treatments a week for several months to rebalance qi energy.

Acupuncture, a cornerstone of many chronic pain clinics, is often utilized when other traditional treatments have not worked.

Acupressure

Acupressure is based on the same principle as acupuncture but the treatment may not be as specific or powerful. The same acupuncture points are stimulated but without a needle and without breaking the skin.

We have discussed the benefits for relieving headaches with acupressure in a previous chapter. Acupressure is also effective for PMS and menstrual cramps. Place two fingers below the belly button and press as you breathe out, then relax the pressure as you inhale. Do for one minute or longer. For back pain associated with menstruation, simultaneously press on both sides of the spine, just below the lowest rib.

Alexander Technique

The Alexander technique teaches the patient to develop a way of supporting the body's weight. It is a process of re-education to improve postural balances and coordination to enable movement with minimum strain and maximum ease. The technique is often used to treat chronic pain, headaches, osteoarthritis, and stress.

Worldwide there are several thousand Alexander teachers. To apply the concept, therapy usually takes 30 lessons of re-education that last 40 to 50 minutes each. One study involving 67 chronic back pain patients found the Alexander technique to improve pain that lasted for six months. There are no risks.

Aroma Therapy

Aroma therapy uses essential oils that can be applied to the skin through massage or a compress. Essential oils can be added to baths, inhaled with steaming water vapor, or sprayed throughout a room. These oils are believed to have both a psychological and physiological effect at the cellular level. In turn, these oils can trigger the limbic system of the brain. Aroma therapy is used to treat headaches, musculoskeletal pain, insomnia, and anxiety.

Ayurvedic Medicine

Ayurvedic medicine is thought to be the oldest medical system in the world. It has an uninterrupted history for thousands of years through the existence of ancient texts that have survived in present time. Today it is practiced alongside modern medicine in India and Sri Lanka. In the United States it was popularized by holistic physician Deepak Chopra, M.D. The Ayurvedic texts describe a wide range of pain syndromes and how to treat them.

The philosophy of Ayurvedic medicine is that all humans can be characterized by their unique mixture of three metabolic types called doshas — vata, pitta, and kapha. Illness occurs if the individual harmony among these three doshas is disturbed, and the aim of Ayurvedic medicine is to insure a balance. The living body functions through these three biofactor principles. Vata is the energetic component composed of all forms of energies including nerve impulses carrying pain. Pitta represents the entire range of the bio-fire system regarding attributes concerning digestion and metabolic activities. Kapha is the component of the body which represents the total solid substance of the organism providing the body with shape and form.

Ayurvedic medicine also emphasizes the need for harmony between body, mind, spirit and the doshas. Any disharmony can be resolved through cleansing, detoxification, palliative, rejuvenation, mental, or spiritual hygiene. Therapy may include herbs, diet, lifestyle, exercise, and massage.

In India there are approximately 300,000 Ayurvedic practitioners and 100 Ayurvedic colleges. Practitioners tend to treat predominantly chronic benign conditions including many pain syndromes. Therapy is usually long term.

Bee Sting Therapy

Bee sting therapy is widely used in Asia, Eastern Europe, and Russia. In the United States it is an underground therapy. A society of beekeepers support and offer this unusual therapy.

Actual bee stings or venom injection by a healer is done on or near the painful area. Bee venom can be given from live bees or by injection of purified bee venom. Injections are usually given by a doctor but this method doesn't seem to be as effective as live bees. For treatment with live bees, the bee is usually grasped with long tweezers and placed on the spot to be stung. Stings can be painful, and one needs many stings or injections to have an effect. If there is no improvement after eight sessions involving a total of 20 to 70 stings, the therapy probably is not working.

Studies show the venom contains powerful anti-inflammatory properties. Thousands of anecdotes claim it relieves arthritis pain. The FDA has approved it to desensitize people with bee allergies. Fatal allergic attacks are always possible but they are rare. It costs $10 for 60 bees to be shipped by mail.

Cannabis (Marijuana)

Marijuana, available by doctor prescription in 24 states and Washington D.C., is used for a variety of health disorders including severe chronic pain, spinal pain, arthritis, headaches, cancer pain, chronic disease, and loss of appetite to name just a few conditions it helps. In the states of Colorado, Washington and Oregon one can purchase marijuana without a prescription. The main active chemical in marijuana is delta-9-tetrahydro cannabinol or THC. THC acts upon specific sites of the brain called cannabinoid receptors.

In 15 of 18 randomized studies, marijuana provided a significant analgesic effect by reducing pain. Marijuana is considered safe and often used only as a second or third option. Possible side effects may include long-term dizzy thinking, memory loss, and possibly cancer.

Cantharidin Plaster

Cantharidin plaster is an application of a chemical skin irritant made out of lytta vesicatoria (Spanish fly) as a form of local pain therapy. Physiologically it promotes the flow of lymph. The technique is used to reduce symptoms of pain therapy for chronic degenerative vertebrae and joint disease, especially in cases of non-operable vertebral disc prolapses. The cantharidin plaster is applied to the painful area and left for 12 to 20 minutes.

Chiropractor Manipulation

Chiropractors are known for their ability to relieve back pain. The profession is concerned with the diagnosis, treatment, and prevention of mechanical disorders of the musculoskeletal system, and the effects of these disorders on the nervous system and general health. Chiropractors believe that pressure on nerves caused by misalignment or subluxation of vertebrae joints can produce disease. By correcting the misalignment, health is regained by relieving nerve pressure. Spinal manipulation often helps joint function and alleviates pain related to spinal abnormalities. Treatment may increase range of motion, alleviate pain, and lengthen the spine. Chiropractors will treat musculoskeletal pain, spinal pain, osteoarthritis, migraines, headaches, asthma, and irritable bowel syndrome. A number of studies have shown chiropractic to be effective.

Colon Therapy

Many arthritis patients have constipation from an accumulation of toxins in the colon and body. Toxins can exacerbate arthritis. Colonic irrigation opens the digestive tract and removes accumulated wastes. When combined with proper diet and supplementation, arthritis may disappear.

Copper Bracelet

According to folklore, wearing a copper bracelet will relieve arthritis pain. To test this folklore, a placebo controlled study was conducted with 300 arthritis patients. Those who wore copper bracelets were compared to a control group who wore bracelets painted to look like copper. Those wearing a copper bracelet had significantly less pain compared to the control group. The copper bracelet group also lost weight. If one is to buy a copper bracelet, it is suggested to buy an inexpensive bracelet that hasn't been treated to prevent tarnishing, so the copper will touch the skin.

Cranial Sacral Therapy

Cranial sacral therapy uses a gentle manipulation to balance the fluids in the craniosacral system that runs from the skull to the base of the spine. The practitioner applies light pressure to the skull. Cranial sacral therapy is practiced by chiropractors, osteopaths, naturopaths, and massage therapists. It is helpful for patients who have chronic pain, headaches, migraines, temporal mandibular disorders, musculoskeletal problems, depression, and more. Some practitioners claim it is helpful in 90 percent of patients, but no studies have confirmed this.

Cupping

Cupping is one of the oldest healing methods used in many different cultures that included ancient Babylonia and Egypt. The healing modality of cupping consists of placing closed cups on predetermined areas of skin that can create a vacuum. The vacuum can be generated by a flame or by suction. This creates a pulling effect on the skin segment that overlays soft tissue and muscle where the pain is located. Cupping draws congestion and pain away from areas buried deep within the body and brings pain closer to the skin surface and eliminates it.

Exercise

Moderate aerobic exercise has been effective for a multitude of pain disorders. Studies have shown it to be effective for headaches, fibromyalgia, knee osteoarthritis, migraine headaches, chronic back pain, peripheral neuropathy, and chronic pain. Pain does not generally get worse over the course of an exercise training program. When exercise is combined with other modalities of pain therapy, there seems to be a greater benefit with these other modalities.

Many studies confirm those who exercise stay healthier, live longer, and cope better with chronic pain. Three disciplines from the ancient East offer alternatives to joint jarring, muscle straining exercises, yet provide many benefits of an athletic workout. These gentle exercises include yoga, tai chi, and qigong. The exercises don't provide an aerobic workout nor the benefit of weight lifting.

Fasting

Therapeutic fasting is an important part of naturopathic pain therapy. Fasting has been found effective in treating pain resulting from rheumatoid arthritis, migraine headaches, and chronic pain.

Therapeutic fasting should take place in a hospital. However, in low grade pain syndromes, outpatient fasting under supervision is often beneficial. A significant improvement in mood is reported by a majority of patients after the third day of fasting. The improvement is maintained through the fasting period. For rheumatoid arthritis, medication should be adjusted during the fast. After four to seven days of fasting, pain relief should be felt. Following the fast, patients should change their eating habits to a semi-vegetarian diet with low arachnoid acids and one that is high in fish oils. During fasting it is easier to reduce analgesic (pain relief) medications. Lifestyle changes should also accompany fasting such as coping strategies for stress, relaxation techniques, etc.

Feldenkrause Technique

The Feldenkrause technique involves the integration of mind and body based on the assumption that improving poor habitual movements will improve self image and health as well as providing symptom relief of pain.

The method is based on a belief that guided exploration of movement promotes attention and awareness of the body. In other words, the method helps one to become aware of the body to explore new movements and skills. Patients are taught exercises for regular home practice. A review of six controlled studies of the Feldenkrause technique found all studies reported positive findings for pain relief of neck, shoulders, and back. Multiple sclerosis patients also reported an improvement in balance.

Forgiveness

Health problems, including pain, can arise because of repressed anger and a lack of forgiveness. Holding on to anger can be destructive to health. Depression and anxiety often underlie anger. To forgive will help release that anger. The art of forgiving implies that one is ready to let go of negative feelings that have affected mind, spirit, and body. People often have no control over the event that caused the anger, but a person does have control over how they react to the event. A positive attitude will prevent a lot of stress, and forgiveness is a good first step. You must also learn to forgive yourself.

Guided Imagery and Visualization

The power of one's imagination can help one cope with many conditions involving pain. With visualization and guided imagery, one can ease pain and anxiety, develop a more positive self-image, and increase the body's healing ability. A practitioner can guide one through various exercises of imagery, or one can practice the technique with help of audio media.

With visualization, one imagines the desired outcome. For example, if one is in pain, one might imagine a place of relaxation or imagine moving about without pain. These techniques of visualization have long been used to control pain.

Sessions, which last 30 to 60 minutes, usually begin with a relaxation meditation or breathing exercise. To relieve pain, one creates a mental image of the symptoms and imagines them melting away, or being swept away from the body. Another technique is to imagine being healthy and going about a loved activity without pain or stress. Studies show visualization can improve the effectiveness of the immune system when combined with other relaxation techniques.

Homeopathy

Homeopathy is often used for chronic pain without any side effects. Homeopathy remedies stimulate self-healing. The homeopathy remedy rhus toxicodendron is often used for pain that is worse at night and pain that occurs in the morning upon awakening. It is also effective against pain that is worse in the cold and damp weather just before a storm.

Hydrotherapy and Balneotherapy

Hydrotherapy is defined as the external application of water in any form or temperature such as hot, cold, steam, liquid, or ice. Balneotherapy is defined as the use of baths with thermal mineral water of at least 68 degrees Fahrenheit and a mineral content of one gram per liter of water. These therapies are often utilized in Europe and frequently reimbursed by health insurance. In Germany, hydrotherapy is part of conventional medicine. It works through physical and chemical stimulation that affects the whole body through the skin. This leads to an adaptive process at the level of muscles, vascular, and metabolic systems. Hydrotherapy is beneficial for back pain, fibromyalgia sufferers, osteoarthritis, and chronic venous insufficiency.

A meta analysis of 230 hydrotherapy studies found back pain benefitted significantly when compared to a control group. Other studies have found improvement in local tenderness and improved rotation of the spine. Most studies have found significant pain improvement in osteoarthritis, fibromyalgia, and rheumatoid arthritis.

Hypnosis

Hypnotherapy involves the induction of a trance-like state to facilitate relaxation, with the goal to gain self-control over behavior, emotions, or physiological processes. Hypnosis is associated with a deep state of relaxation, often used for pain, psychosomatic conditions, post traumatic stress syndrome (PTSD), anxiety, and phobias. There are good scientific studies showing its effectiveness.

A meta-analysis of studies regarding pain management report a moderate to large effect in reducing pain. Controlled studies have found it reduces chronic pain and osteoarthritis pain when compared to a control group. Hypnosis is also effective for headaches, child birth pain, irritable bowel syndrome, fibromyalgia, fatigue, stress, and burn pain.

Immersion in Water

A review of eight controlled studies of pregnant women who used any kind of bath tub or pool use during the first stage of labor experienced reduced pain and need for analgesics when compared to a control group without immersion.

Laser Therapy

Laser therapy is often used for musculoskeletal injuries, chronic and degenerating conditions, and for healing wounds. The light source is placed on the skin allowing photon energy to penetrate tissue. Studies found it to be effective for neck pain, rheumatoid arthritis, and chronic low back pain. Laser therapy should be considered for short term or chronic pain conditions.

Laser Therapy (Low Energy)

Low energy laser light, also called cold laser, is often used for soft tissue injuries. It emits gentle energy that can penetrate deep into the tissue without damage. Laser therapy is thought to increase circulation, relieve inflammation, and reduce pain. Low energy lasers are used in musculoskeletal conditions, osteoarthritis, rheumatoid arthritis, fibromyalgia, carpel tunnel syndrome, strains, and soft tissue injuries. A typical treatment lasts five minutes in a series of fifteen sessions. The technique is not FDA approved.

A review of 36 randomized clinical trials involving 1704 patients found low energy laser therapy was significantly better than a placebo. Rheumatoid arthritis sufferers benefitted from it. Another study found it reversed carpel tunnel syndrome symptoms in 77 percent of 30 people treated.

Many acupuncture doctors have used cold lasers instead of needles. Lasers can stimulate acupuncture points, reduce muscle spasms, and move qi energy. One should not point the laser directly at the heart, eyes, or Adam's apple.

Leech Therapy

The medical leech was described by ancient Greece nearly 2,200 years ago. In Germany, there are approximately 350,000 leeches that are farmed for medical therapy, including various types of pain syndromes. Leeches have been effective for chronic pain and osteoarthritis, especially effective for the knee. To treat knee arthritis, four to six leeches are placed each day on the skin of the knee. When applied to the skin, they bite, suck blood, and secrete saliva. After sucking enough blood they will drop off. If correctly used, there are no side effects.

One study involved 51 knee osteoarthritis patients using leech therapy who were compared to a control group using the pain drug diclofenac. Leech therapy was superior in reducing pain.

Light Emission Diodes (LED)

LED therapy is used to treat muscle pain and joint stiffness associated with arthritis. LED therapy is used by NASA and by the U.S. submarine fleet. The FDA has approved LED light therapy for the treatment of minor pain. Light waves of 880 NM go deep into muscle tissue to stimulate DNA production, and promote cell growth.

Massage

Massage therapy is among the most utilized of all the complementary therapies. It is the manipulation of soft tissue using pressure and traction, often used for back pain, musculoskeletal conditions, depression, anxiety, stress, and many other conditions. Massage will free the flow of vital energy so that the painful area of the body may benefit from healthy blood circulation. There are more than 100 various types of body work, with studies showing massage effective for many conditions including pain.

Swedish massage emphasizes the physical by using pressure, rubbing, and manipulation to work on muscles, joints, and improved function. Swedish massage is effective for muscles spasms by improving circulation.

Asian massage techniques emphasizes the balancing of vital energy flow in the body. Thai massage uses stretching, while Japanese shiatsu and Chinese tui are deep and often painful.

Reiki and therapeutic touch will focus energy for spiritual healing. Practitioners don't physically touch the body.

Trigger point therapy uses deep pressure on specific spots to release trigger point pain in other parts of the body.

Reflexology therapy uses massage points on the feet, hands, or ears that correspond to organs in other parts of the body. A placebo controlled study on 38 women with PMS who received reflexology were compared to women who received a sham treatment. The reflexology group reported significantly fewer symptoms.

Studies have shown massage to help with fibromyalgia by relieving pain and depression and improving life quality. Massage has been shown to provide pain relief and psychic support during labor. It also has been proven beneficial for postoperative pain by reducing symptoms. Studies have shown it to be effective for shoulder pain, neck pain, and chronic low back pain.

Magnets

Research has shown that magnets are effective in relieving pain for osteoarthritis, rheumatoid arthritis, neuropathy, fibromyalgia, and knee pain. Magnets come in all sizes and shapes, but no one knows how these magnets work to relieve pain. Some people hypothesize magnets increase circulation; some believe they suppress inflammation; some think that perhaps they affect C-fiber pain transmission; and others believe they change the polarization of cells. Magnets are usually placed on the body over the pain area, or in the soles of shoes, or in seat covers, and even in mattress pads. The strength of therapy magnets range from 300 to 4,000 gauss.

Animal studies found a 3,000 gauss magnet can decrease inflammation levels. A double blind magnet study involving post-polio pain subjects found 76 percent had decreased pain compared to 19 percent in a control group. Another study involved 20 people with peripheral foot neuropathy caused by poor circulation. Magnets significantly reduced pain in 90 percent of the subjects compared to 30 percent of the placebo group.

Meditation

Meditation is a relaxation technique that can be of various forms including repeating a mantra, listening to the breath, detaching from the thought process, or a self-directed mental practice, all with the purpose of achieving an inner calm.

Numerous studies have shown that relaxation can relieve pain, with research demonstrating that meditation can change physiological parameters such as oxygen consumption respiration rate, and brain function. Meditation can relieve anxiety, stress, asthma, hypertension, and heart disease. Over 800 studies have been done regarding transcendental meditation. One such study demonstrated that meditation can relieve low back pain and the psychological distress accompanying it.

Moxibustion

Moxibustion therapy is utilized in Chinese medicine to relieve pain. It involves burning mugwort herb over acupuncture points.

Music Therapy

Music therapy has been evaluated for pain relief in 51 studies involving a variety of pain syndromes. It is frequently used for chronic pain. Studies have found listening to music reduces pain levels by an average of 0.5 on a 10 point scale and increased the likelihood of 50 percent pain relief in 70 percent of postoperative patients. Opioid requirements were also reduced. One controlled study found it significantly reduced chronic osteoarthritis pain in an elderly community, while another study found music therapy to be beneficial for labor pain.

Myotherapy

Myotherapy involves trigger points which are found in muscle tissue that has been hurt or damaged. Trigger points can lie quiet in muscles but when there is a physical and/or emotional stress, they come to life and one experiences pain. Essentially a trigger point is a highly irritable spot in a muscle and contributes to pain when activated by throwing the muscle into spasm. The major causes of trigger points include birth, accidents, sports, occupation, and disease.

To find a trigger point, press down with your fingers/hand on the tissue. If there is a tenderness verging on pain, you have found a trigger point. Hold that pressure for seven seconds and then slowly release the pressure. You can do myotherapy over several days, perhaps three minutes a day. If an area is very sensitive, you can bring more pressure in following sessions. The first session is the most painful, but it gets easier.

In summary, you can do myotherapy on yourself by:

1. Locating the trigger point.
2. Apply seven seconds of pressure to where it hurts.
3. Then stretch the affected muscle with simple exercise.

Myotherapy is used on people of all ages. It is safe, long term, and provides pain relief for arthritis, backaches, headaches, menstrual cramps, tennis elbow, trick knees, bursitis, and many more conditions. *Prevention* magazine states, "The amazing thing is that it works." Clinical trials show it is effective about 95 percent of the time.

Naturopathy

A naturopath physician (N.D.) is a health care professional involved in an eclectic array of healing modalities that incorporate both complementary and conventional medicine to enhance the self healing process. The philosophy underlying naturopathy is that health can be influenced by nature's own healing power, with the idea illness is a result of violating general principles underlying a healthy lifestyle. Naturopaths use natural remedies to relieve pain.

Ordnungs Therapy

Ordnungs therapy is one of five cornerstones of Kneipp's classic naturopathy, which also includes nutrition, herbs, exercise, and water therapy. Patients receive instructions on a number of self-help strategies regarding nutrition, exercise, and relaxation from specially trained mind-body instructors and physicians. The permanent lifestyle changes may include yoga, qigong, and meditation. In order to achieve long term relief, it is important that patients practice these techniques 20-45 minutes daily, as well as integrate relaxation and mindfulness into these daily routines.

Studies confirm the effectiveness of Ordnungs therapy for chronic pain, fibromyalgia, breast cancer pain, chronic headaches, and rheumatic diseases.

Osteopathy

Osteopathy is a form of manual therapy performed by an osteopath (D.O.) involving the manipulation of soft tissue and peripheral and spinal joints. Osteopaths mostly treat patients suffering from musculoskeletal problems, especially back and neck pain. Scientific studies suggest that osteopathy is helpful for low back pain. Sadly, most American osteopaths no longer use manipulation techniques routinely.

Physiatry

A physiatrist is a medical doctor who specializes in a branch of medicine that uses modalities such as heat, light, water, and electricity to diagnose, treat, and prevent a wide array of physical problems. Their goal is to reduce pain and restore the normal function and movement of the body. Often physiatrists work with physical therapists, occupational therapists, psychiatrists, nurses and other health practitioners to help relieve pain. Some view the physiatrists as a coach. There are approximately 4,000 physiatrists in the United States.

Physical Therapists

Physical therapists use technology and their own two hands to treat a wide variety of pain problems ranging from sprained muscles, whip lash, accident injuries, cancer pain, and postsurgical pain.

Physical therapists may use exercise programs, traction, ultrasound, heat and cold to help relieve pain. Often patients will choose physical therapy over surgery to relieve pain. Manual manipulation and massage play an important role in physical therapy, which often leads to relief of pain and stiffness in muscles, soft tissue, and skeletal disorders. Patients are often given a set of exercises to help relieve the pain. Exercise is the most effective way of getting blood flow to the pain area. Both stretching and strengthening exercises are beneficial, and can be done at home.

Ultrasound therapy often used by physical therapists, involves high frequency sound waves to heat the deep tissue of the muscles, which can raise temperature by 5 degrees. Traction involves a pulling force on the skeletal structure to relieve pain.

Phytotherapy (Herbology)

Western phytotherapy consists of using plants to prevent, relieve, and heal diseases. It is also known as herbology, discussed in earlier chapters. Certain plants have healing properties whether it be from the leaves, flowers, or roots. Phytotherapy is one of the five cornerstones of Kneipp's classic naturopathy, which includes nutrition, exercise, water therapy, and Ordnungs therapy. Preparation extracts from plants may be in the form of pills or tea. Herbal preparations are primarily indicated in mild to moderate pain. Studies have shown herbal remedies can reduce the intake of NSAID drugs.

Platelet Rich Plasma Injection (PRP)

Platelet rich plasma injections uses the patients own blood platelets to repair tissue damage, to accelerate healing from injuries and surgery. Dr. Alan Lazer, M.D., in his book *Beyond the Knife: Alternatives to Surgery* details his procedure of medical injections to relieve pain and repair damaged tissue such as cartilage destroyed by osteoarthritis, torn tendons, and damaged ligaments.

PRP is an in-office procedure where the doctor removes a minimal amount of patient's blood stem cells and fat, and then injects the combined fluid into the injured area or arthritic joint. The bioactive tissue growth factors are released when the platelets are injected into the injured area. This stimulates a healing cascade for musculoskeletal injuries and arthritis. Remarkable results have been reported for regeneration of cartilage in osteoarthritis of thumbs, knees, and hips. PRP is not approved by Medicare or insurance companies.

Posturology

Most people have some irregularity in their posture which may cause pain over time. Good posture is important because it prevents chronic pain from developing as a result of poor circulation. Paul St. John teaches a course on posture in a pain clinic in Clearwater, FL regarding:

1. Eliminating muscle spasm
2. Restoring flexibility
3. Restoring proper biomechanics
4. Increasing muscle strength
5. Increasing muscle endurance

Pulsed Electromagnetic Field Therapy (PEMF)

Pulsed electromagnetic field therapy is medically accepted for treatment of some pain conditions such as osteoarthritis. The technique has been used successfully for healing broken bones. In Europe it is widely accepted for treating osteoarthritis but has not been approved in the United States. Controlled studies have shown it to relieve pain in knee osteoarthritis. It is believed that PEMF stimulates repair by replacing a short circuit in the normal electrical process of the body. Low level doses of external electrical stimulus may signal the body to repair cartilage.

The person is placed inside a circular magnetic device that looks like a doughnut, where an electrical current creates a pulsed electromagnetic field. Treatment is painless, and studies show it relieves pain and improves function. A study of 18 osteoarthritis patients at Yale University found those who received treatment had up to 61 percent improvement in reducing pain and joint tenderness compared to 18 percent in the placebo group. A study at Johns Hopkins University was conducted on 78 subjects with knee osteoarthritis over four weeks. The treatment group had a significant reduction in pain and improved function compared to the placebo group. PEMF has been used effectively for carpel tunnel syndrome.

Qigong

Qigong is an ancient Asian art that uses gentle, focused exercise for the mind and body to increase and restore the flow of qi energy (life force energy) for the purpose of accelerating the healing process. Qigong involves five steps for healing that include meditation, cleansing, recharging, strengthening, and circulation of qi. Each one of the steps comprise specific exercises, meditation, and sounds. Qigong consists of two main protocols involving controlled deep breathing with slow body movement, and aerobic exercise combined with relaxation.

Studies have shown qigong to be effective for reducing pain in fibromyalgia, shoulder and arm pain, regional pain syndrome, breast cancer pain, and PMS pain.

Reflexology

Reflexology is a therapeutic healing modality utilizing manual pressure applied to specific zones on the feet, hands or ears. Foot reflexology is the most common practice. Each zone on the foot corresponds to other areas of the body, including organs and glands. Reflexologists believe that the health of the body can be assessed by examining the feet to detect an imbalance of qi energy, which is expressed as tenderness. By massaging the tender area, the organ or corresponding body part will be relieved of pain or symptoms.

Reflexology has been found to relieve pain, reduce stress, improve circulation, eliminate toxins, and promote metabolic homeostasis. It has been effective in helping various pain syndromes such as arthritis, back and neck pain, migraine headaches, tension headaches, chronic fatigue, digestive problems, irritable bowel syndrome, and many other stress maladies.

Reiki

Reiki involves a spiritually guided universal life energy, with no contact between practitioner and patient. Energy is transmitted from practitioner's hands to the patient. Reiki has been found effective for relieving symptoms in chronic disease, arthritis, lupus, and other pain syndromes.

Relaxation Therapy

Relaxation therapy as discussed in earlier chapters has been found to be effective for many pain syndromes. It elicits a relaxation response of the autonomic nervous system. Progressive muscle relaxation is based on the premise that it is impossible to be tense in any part of the body where the muscles are completely relaxed. Studies have shown that relaxation techniques are beneficial for headaches, anxiety, depression, ischemic pain, migraine headaches, cancer pain, menopausal pain, and rheumatoid arthritis. Relaxation modalities include biofeedback, hypnotherapy, and meditation.

Rolfing

Rolfing is a technique similar to deep tissue massage which releases fascia tightness cased by injuries, stress, and misuse. Rolfing has been effective for pain conditions including arthritis. Weekly one hour treatments are usually spread over ten weeks.

Shiatsu

This Japanese therapy involves applying pressure mainly with the finger or hand to certain parts of the body. Shiatsu views health as being a state of balance which is maintained by the flow of life energy along specific meridians. A disease is believed to occur when the energy flow is blocked, deficient, or is in excess. Shiatsu restores the normal energy flow and has been shown to be effective for musculoskeletal conditions, psychological problems, neck pain, shoulder pain, lower back pain, arthritis, depression, and anxiety.

Spiritual Healing

Spiritual healers believe the therapeutic effect from their healing comes from channeling of healing energy from a higher source by way of the healer to the patient. A review of 23 placebo controlled studies found half of the studies showed a positive effect for spiritual healing. There have also been many studies confirming the power of prayer and healing.

Stem Cell (Amniotic) Therapy

Stem cell therapy may be the next big health care advancement in non-surgical pain management. Many consider it to be the medicine of the future. The procedure for amniotic stem cell therapy for pain was discovered in 2007, and research began in 2011 to explore its many potentials for pain management and other attributes.

Stem cells are natural cells found in the body that are responsible for healing damaged joints, cartilage, and muscles. The body is constantly rebuilding the damaged tissue with the help of stem cells. After the age of 40, the number of stem cells and their potency significantly decrease each year. This explains why a 21-year-old person can heal much faster than a 65-year-old.

Stem cells used at pain clinics are called "amniotic stem cells," which come from the amniotic sac, not from embryos. Amniotic stem cells are harvested from a donating mother during a scheduled c-section, and then processed at an FDA approved lab. The cells are rigorously tested like other biological tissue before they are sent to pain clinics. The use of amniotic stem cells raises no moral issues, unlike embryo stem cells. Amniotic stem cells are 'neutral cells' that contain no DNA. Because of this neutrality, patients cannot have a rejection or reaction to them. They are completely safe. Since 2007, there has not been an adverse effect documented in the tens of thousand procedures.

Amniotic stem cells can turn into almost any type of tissue because they just grew a baby. They are brand new cells which are extremely potent, meaning they can heal tissue very quickly in most parts of the body. For example, a patient may have meniscus damage in the joint, a frayed ligament, weak tendons, and minor fracture of the bone. Amniotic stem cells have the ability to heal all those structures.

Amniotic stem cells are reported to have natural anti-inflammatory and pain relieving properties that are more effective than steroids. Pain clinics report the majority of patients leave the clinic with little or no pain by the time the analgesic wears off. For example, knee tissue has healed enough so there is no longer pain.

A pain-score study conducted on 200 patients at the Pain MD Clinic in Coeur d'Alene, Idaho found that before treatment, the average pain score was 7.7 on a scale of one to ten. After one month, the average pain score was 3.1. After 27 months, the clinical improvement held. In 95 percent of the cases, only one procedure was required. The results are even better when combined with Platelet Rich Plasma Therapy.

The procedure takes less than 20 minutes, which involves injection into the painful area. It often heals other parts of the body. Clinical findings have found amniotic stem cell therapy is effective for osteoarthritis, rheumatoid arthritis, back pain, neuropathy, fibromyalgia, erectile dysfunction, Alzheimer's disease, Parkinson's disease, multiple sclerosis, thyroid conditions, cancer, visual disturbances, macular degeneration, and many more conditions.

Stem cell therapy has been effective for diabetic neuropathy because it can grow new blood vessels and nerves. Relief comes in four weeks. There have been 45 clinical studies involving 1,272 patients. It prevents amputation.

At this time insurance companies and medicare do not cover stem cell therapy. The price at the Pain MD Clinic in Coeur d'Alene, Idaho is about $6,500. For a free consultation call (208) 667-7246. Their website is www.idpainmd.com.

Another stem cell clinic for pain is located in northern Colorado at the Premier Stem Cell Institute. Call (866) 647-9405 for a free consultation.

Support Groups

Chronic pain often makes people depressed, fearful, angry, hopeless, and lonely. When people meet with others undergoing a similar situation there is a healing value in sharing experiences. Support groups come together to help each other and share problems. Some support groups are therapeutic, often led by a counselor, psychotherapist, or social worker. Support groups are offered through pain clinics or rehabilitation hospitals. It is an opportunity for one to express feelings and learn coping skills to assist in recovering. Support groups encourage pain sufferers to do all things they want to do, perhaps on a limited basis. It is a place for information exchange, which may help people obtain better medical treatment. There are several national organizations regarding pain support groups including:

1. The American Chronic Pain Association, which has over 13,000 members and 450 chapters around the country, the largest network for chronic pain support groups.
2. The Chronic Pain Support Groups
3. The Natural Chronic Pain Outreach Association

   Check the internet for current contact information.

Tai Chi

Tai chi, originating from ancient Chinese philosophy and martial arts, is an exercise involving movements and postures to enhance mental and physical health. It is based on the principle of two opposing forces, yin and yang. Ill health is considered to be an imbalance between yin (female energy) and yang (male energy). A review of nine controlled studies found tai chi to be effective for both physiological and psychological functions. It is safe and promotes good balance. Research has demonstrated tai chi to be effective for rheumatoid arthritis and osteoarthritis patients.

Traditional Chinese Medicine (TCM)

Chinese medicine believes everything in nature consists of two opposing forces, ying (female energy) and yang (male energy). Disease results in the loss of relative balance between ying and yang. Traditional Chinese medicine believes there are meridians in the body that allow qi energy to circulate. The meridians permit communication between various internal organs. Pain results when the flow of qi is interrupted. Chronic pain results when the body's immune system is weaker than the pain promoting system. TCM believes pain is caused by five factors:

1. Externally by six climatic excesses
2. Internal damage to the seven emotions
3. Phlegm and stagnation of the blood
4. Lifestyle problems such as diet and exercise
5. Trauma and infectious disorders

The Chinese believe that each type of inappropriate management of emotion may lead to pain. For example, worry can block qi energy while joy relaxes qi energy. Pain results if there is an obstruction of qi energy and flow of blood. Obstruction of qi flow and blood flow play a role in either acute or chronic pain.

Treatment promotes qi flow and blood movement. In traditional Chinese medicine, there are four specific treatments to relieve pain including acupuncture, moxibustion, cupping, and herbs. To prevent pain, TCM recommends:

1. Control strong emotions
2. Regular physical exercise
3. Adequate nutrition
4. Balanced lifestyle
5. Avoid pathogenic factors

Therapeutic Touch

Therapeutic touch is based on the theory that we all have an energy field beyond our physical body. By entering a meditative state, a practitioner uses his or her hands to feel problems in the patients energy field. The practitioner then channels universal energy through his or her hands to help disease and pain. It is a popular healing modality often used by nurses and is taught in over 80 universities. A 1998 therapeutic study conducted on 25 patients with osteoarthritis demonstrated a significant reduction in pain and improved function compared to a control group.

Thermal Therapy

A common treatment for pain is thermal therapy involving the application of heat and cold by various means such as hot packs, cold packs, paraffin wax, baths, and faradic baths. Positive results for rheumatoid arthritis have been achieved with paraffin wax, which has helped with better range of motion and grip strength following four weeks of treatment.

Balneotherapy, spa therapy, was found to show positive results in six studies for pain relief and improved joint function in rheumatoid arthritis patients. For osteoarthritis of the knee, studies have shown ice massage reduced swelling, improved range of motion, and knee strength. Heat wrap therapy for low back pain has been found to provide short term pain relief.

Transcutaneous Electrical Nerve Stimulation (TENS)

One of the most often prescribed pain remedies that is not a pill or injection is TENS. TENS units provide a tiny electrical current supplied by electrodes taped to the skin. As a result, pain messages traveling to the brain are jammed, interfering with pain signals trying to reach the brain. One or more of the electrodes are placed directly over the pain site, or over a nerve leading to the pain site, or over an acupuncture point near the pain. TENS units generally provide pain relief only when it is being used and for a short time afterward. A 'pins and needle' sensation is experienced during TENS treatment.

Another form of stimulation is called 'acupuncture-like TENS.' The current is strong and slow as compared to the conventional TENS therapy. Most TENS units have both conventional and acupuncture settings.

TENS units are popular because they are easy to use with little risk. A variety of TENS units is available, with some providers advertising for menstrual cramps and some for arthritis. They have been used for all types of pain.

Many studies have been done on TENS. A University of Colorado Medical School study found at least half of patients had an initial positive result with TENS. Other studies demonstrate the initial good response fell off dramatically during the first year with only 30 percent still having satisfactory results. With stronger stimulation, a small number of chronic pain patients remain comfortable for years. Patients who use the TENS units after surgery require fewer pain killers. In Scandinavia, TENS units are used for childbirth without side effects, with 10 percent of women not requiring pain medication.

In the United States, TENS is most often prescribed for pain lasting for six months or more. It is often prescribed to reduce pain medication. TENS is most frequently used for back pain, and also recommended for rheumatoid arthritis, osteoarthritis, diabetic neuropathy, knee and hip pain, and some cancer pain. Treatment by TENS is often limited to six months. One can buy a TENS unit for about $500 or rent one. Medicare and insurance will pay up to 80 percent of the costs.

True Pulse A 2000 (Pulsed Electromagnetic Field)

Pulsed Electromagnetic Field Energy (PEMF) was studied by NASA, which found that a magnetic field was essential to maintain the health of astronauts in space. They found a pulsing magnetic field assisted the body in healing itself. As the PEMF was introduced to the public, its broad spectrum healing and pain relief capabilities became apparent.

Pulsed Harmonix, based in Longmont, Colorado, has introduced a highly effective state of the art machine called the "True Pulse A 2000." The technology used to produce the pulse has been classified as "space technology." Over 70 percent of the hundreds of volunteers who have been tested report measurable pain relief within one 15 to 30 minute session. Amazingly, more than one half of the volunteers reported their pain was relieved in that one session.

The pulsed electromagnetic field device uses electrical energy to direct a series of magnetic pulses through the body, blood cells, organs, muscles, bones, and brain. Each magnetic pulse induces a strong reaction in the body that detoxifies and rejuvenates at the same time. The True Pulse A 2000 can be used for long-term therapy sessions with no risk of adverse effects. It is registered as an FDA Class 1 Medical device.

The device is highly portable, about the size of a shoe box, weighing only 4.6 pounds. It runs on 120 volt household AC current plus a special 180 watt, 12 volt inverter, making it an exceptional healing and energizing companion while on long trips. It can be used when working, driving, and sleeping. The True Pulse delivers a wide range of harmonic frequencies, combined with a broad range of power settings to maintain optimal health.

After Nobel Laureate Linus Pauling was introduced to PEMF technology, he said "PEMF is a benefit for mankind from infant to geriatric. PEMF will lead to a change in the paradigm of medicine." Research conducted by leading government and university research facilities has consistently demonstrated that PEMF has wide-spectrum healing effects on virtually any adverse condition of humans and animals. A series of non-controlled studies found the True Pulse A 2000 reduced pain by an average of 51 percent in a single session of 15 to 30 minutes. Another study involving 331 subjects found the average pain reduction was 83 percent. Overall, 72 percent of the 331 subjects experienced pain relief from 40 to 100 percent.

The cost of True Pulse A 2000 complete system is $2,800, with a 30 day full money back guaranteed less a $200 restocking fee. Orders can be placed at the company's website at www.Pulsedharmonix.com or by calling (855) 749-7363.

Ultrasound Therapy

Therapeutic ultrasound is often used by physical therapists for the management of chronic pain and loss of function.

Pain Pen and Pain Pad

These recently developed pain relief devices by the Kesche Foundation in Europe appear to be very effective for pain relief according to many anecdotal reports. The pain pen is designed to reduce inflammation and help regenerate tissue. Also called the plasma pen, it generates nano particles from its copper coils creating nano copper oxide that causes a plasma field to be directed down the pen. This plasma field interacts with the cellular plasma field allowing it to regenerate into a natural state. One can also point the pen towards a glass of water causing it to pick up the plasma pattern from other sources. Some researchers believe it can pattern food nutrients into the water. The technology is based on magnetic/gravitational fields that penetrate 3 cm into the tissue affecting the plasma/matter state. Developed by M.T. Kesche, a nuclear engineer from Europe, who has also developed a free energy device. They sell for 35 Euros and 45 Euros respectively. Google Kesche Foundation to order. Toroid Systems will be manufacturing the plasma pen in the United States in the near future. (Google Toroid Systems once they have them in production.) This new technology may revolutionize health care according to the many successful testimonials.

Yoga

The purpose of yoga is to join the mind, body, and spirit in harmonious relaxation. For over 3,000 years, yoga has been practiced by Hindis in India. Yoga is believed to increase the flow of vital energy, called 'prana' in India and 'qi' in China. A poor diet, stress, and other lifestyle factors are believed to block the natural flow of prana. A large survey in the United Kingdom found yoga to be the most satisfying of all alternative modalities. Controlled studies have found yoga therapy to be effective for back pain, carpel tunnel syndrome, and reduced joint stiffness in osteoarthritis.

There are other natural pain remedies, but the ones discussed in this book have some science that gives them credibility. It is up to the patient to take responsibility for his or her health and find the pain remedy that is most effective and safe for him or her, which may be through trial and error. Because this is a book about natural therapies, one might use the technique of applied kinesiology (muscle testing) to help determine the most effective therapy or by dowsing with the pendulum. (See appendix II for guidelines.) Good luck in finding a natural remedy that works for you!

APPENDIX I

Various Commercial Remedies

The following is a list of alternative pain therapies gathered from advertisements found on television commercials, magazines, and newspapers in recent years. Most are based on alternatives discussed in this book. Contact information is given regarding the product. (The author is not receiving any reimbursement for mentioning products.)

Arthritis

1. **Arthopure:** FDA approved supplement. Some doctors recommend this before using NSAIDs. Call (888) 941-4890.
2. **Hyalgan:** FDA approved. Hyalgan is made from the extraction of hyaluronic acid of rooster combs. Hyalgan is injected into knee joints for three to five treatments over one month. According to Michael Axe, M.D., clinical professor at the University of Delaware, 75 percent of 15,000 patients have improved symptoms within five injections. Osteo Relief Institute, Denver, CO, (303) 952-4469.
3. **Instaflex:** This supplement contains glucosamine, turmeric, white willow bark, hyaluronic acid, and boswellia serrata. It is advertised to improve pain, mobility, flexibility, and joint lubrication. It was studied by North Carolina Research Campus. Instaflex is available at vitamin stores, GNC, Vitamin Shoppe, Walgreens, CVS, and Rite Aid.
4. **SemperFlex:** This supplement claims to be more effective than glucosamine/chondroitin. It is advertised in Health Science Institute literature. (800) 817-2575.

5. **Joint Flex:** The remedy contains camphor, glucosamine, and chondroitin sulfate. Joint Flex is a nonprescription pain relieving cream. Studies have shown substantial pain relief after application. One study found the majority of subjects obtained long-term pain relief that continued throughout the entire eight-week study. www.jointflex.com. (800) 411-7917.
6. **Arthritis Relief Cream:** The cream gets rid of arthritis pain in 30 minutes, according to Allan Spreen, M.D. It is advertised in Health Science Institute literature. (888) 213-0764.
7. **Ostinol:** This medicinal formula works to ease pain by decreasing the inflammatory markers interleukin 1 and interleukin 6. Ostinol contains the only proteins proven to activate stem cells that stimulate new bone and cartilage growth. These proteins accelerate the healing process in bones and joints. Ostinol seems to actually help repair damaged joints in osteoarthritis as well as relieving the pain. Several controlled studies have found Ostinol to be very effective for reducing pain without side effects.

    Ostinol comes in three dosages - 150 mg, 350 mg, and 450 mg. It is safe to take 900 mg daily. The cost is $45 for one bottle of 150 mg capsules and $109 for a bottle of 450 mg capsules. Zycal Bioceuticals manufactures Ostinol, which can be ordered by calling (888) 779-9225 or at www.zylcalbio.com. Mention HSI (Health Science Institute) when you order and receive a discount.
8. **Sun Chorella:** Research shows this remedy blocks the cox-2 enzyme to relieve pain. One study found 70 percent experienced improved comfort. www.sunhealthspecial.com.
9. **Synerflex:** Synerflex contains boron, boswellia, and hylajoint. It is advertised in Health Science Institute literature. (800) 537-9687.
10. **Joint Performance Plus:** This remedy contains UC-II collagen, turmeric, grape seed extract, ginger root powder, pomegranate extract, and MSM. It is advertised in Health Science Institute literature. (800) 818-1251.

11. **Oxyrub:** One double blind study found Oxyrub decreased pain by 28 percent and improved mobility and flexibility by 60 percent by creating hyper oxygenation to the painful tissue. Oxyrub is effective for arthritis and bursitis. (800) 963-1053.
12. **Apple Cider Vinegar and Honey:** This remedy has been touted as a cure for chronic pain of arthritis. Mix a tablespoon of honey and a tablespoon of apple cider vinegar into a warm glass of water. Take daily.
13. **Curamin:** Curamin is a pain formula derived from timeless herbs including curcumin and boswellia. Curamin is advertised to impact every inflammatory pathway in the body including leukotrines, 5-LOX, cox-1, and cox-2. Curamin is known to knock out pain without negative side effects including joint pain, nerve pain, and trauma. Controlled studies have found it to be effective for osteoarthritis. A recent study found it to be as effective as ibuprofen for osteoarthritis knee pain. Clinical studies have found it to be safe and effective for rheumatoid arthritis, osteoarthritis, colitis, and Crohn's disease. When boswellia and curcumin work together, they are more effective than Celebrex. The manufacturer recommends taking one Curamin capsule up to three times a day with food. The cost is $38.95 for 60 capsules. Call (877) 575-5755 or go to www.TerryNaturallyVitamins.com.

Multiple Pain Disorders

1. **Oil of Eucalyptus:** The oil soothes and penetrates the skin to bring quick relief to arthritic and rheumatic sufferers. It is effective for back pain, knee pain, carpel tunnel syndrome, gout, and more. Janco, FL (727) 937-1364, NY (607) 498-5788.
2. **Cold Laser Therapy:** Cold laser therapy is used for neuropathy, carpel tunnel syndrome, sciatic back pain, headaches, and herniated disc. Rocky Mountain Spine and Disc, John Smith, D.C., (970) 682-2667.

3. **Soothanal XL:** This supplement is advertised to have instant pain relief. Ingredients include menthol, capsaicin, wintergreen, calendula oil, ginger, arnica, orange peel extract, virgin olive oil, and St. John's Wort. It has been used by 500,000 pain sufferers without any media advertising. It is advertised in Health Science Institute literature. (800) 537-9687.
4. **Omega XL:** This remedy is advertised to heal pain and inflammation naturally. (800) 894-7148.
5. **Painwizard:** The cream remedy contains 20 healing ingredients, manufactured in Colorado. wwwpainwizard.com.
6. **Rezil:** Listed with the FDA. Rezil is a topical pain relieving lotion that relieves pain from arthritis, tendinitis, bursitis, neuralgia, sprains, and strains. It contains capsaicin which blocks pain signals. Toqara, Denver, CO (303) 205-9032, (855) 697-3945.
7. **Eucalyptus Essential Oil:** This essential oil for pain relief can be purchased at www.institutefornaturalhealingcom.
8. **Pets:** Pets have been found to improve pain, mood, and distress. www.petpartners.com.
9. **Zyflamend**: This anti-inflammatory supplement contains six herbs that include rosemary, turmeric, and oregano.
10. **Oregano:** This herb/spice can alleviate osteoarthritis symptoms and other inflammatory conditions. Oregano has dozens of anti-inflammatory compounds that act as muscle relaxants and pain relievers. Oregano protects the heart by helping to prevent clots and irregular heart rhythms. Oregano can be purchased at health food stores.

Headaches

1. **Denver Headache Center:** The headache center helps people with chronic headaches, TMJ, jaw pain, tinnitus, and vertigo. Patients are provided with an at-home care kit. Dr. Charles Barotz claims a 95 percent success rate. denverheadachecenter.com, (303) 595-4994.

Neuropathy

1. **Nerve Shield:** This remedy contains herbs and nutrients such as turmeric, barkal skullcap, alpha lipsic acid, and B vitamins. It is advertised in Health Science Institute literature. (888) 453-5058.
2. **MagniLife Diabetic Neuropathy Foot Cream:** The foot cream is available at Walgreens and Rite Aid. www.MDfootcream.com, (800) 659-3015.

Digestion

1. **Aloecure:** This supplement is used for digestive problems, heartburn, acid-reflux, constipation, gas, bloating, and diarrhea, with over 14 million bottles sold. (855) 614-7205.

Sciatica

1. **MagniLife Sciatica Relief:** The remedy is available at CVS, Walgreens, and Rite Aid. www.magnilife.com or (800) 516-3481. The ad reads, "If you suffer from sciatica symptoms such as intense pain in the buttocks and lower back, or pain and numbness in your legs and feet, you are not alone. Over 170 million people suffer from burning, tingling, numbing, and shooting pains because they are not aware of this proven treatment."

Fibromyalgia

1. **NT Factor:** This supplement is a vibrant and clear-energy wafer. It is advertised in Health Science Institute literature. (800) 950-0387.
2. **SHINE:** SHINE stands for sleep, hormones, infection, natural supplements, and exercise. This supplement benefits about 90 percent of patients with fibromyalgia.
3. **Magnilife Fibromyalgia Relief:** This remedy has been specifically formulated for fibromyalgia patients. It combines 11 active ingredients including coniium. It is available at CVS and Rite Aid. (800) 730-4173.

Pain Devices

1. **Pain Relieving Neuromuscular Stimulator System:** This is a TENS unit that sells for $129.95. (800) 543-3366.
2. **Copper Hands:** These are gloves worn for arthritis. Two sets sell for $12.99. (800) 560-0131.
3. **The Triple Therapy Knee Pain Reliever:** The pain device combines LED (light emission diode) therapy, vibration, and compression massage. It fits around the knee, so is hands free. (800) 543-3366.
4. **Frequency Band:** The frequency band is worn all the time. It is thought to release endorphins, to reduce pain, numbness, and stinging. Money-back guarantee. NGBalance.com. (615) 497-0094, (615) 497-0099.
5. **Soleve:** This device is used for back pain. The non-invasive machine scans the body and prints out a chart that shows the primary pain areas. It is very precise involving a two-minute electrified stimulant that then moves to the next painful area. Therapy usually involves five treatments. Some chiropractors use this device. Florida (813) 978-0020.
6. **Dr. Ho's Decompression Back Belt:** This device is used for chronic back pain. It can help leg pain caused by degenerating discs and sleep disorders due to back pain. The belt pumps up and expands to decompress the pressure and provides support to help relieve pain. Medicare covers the belt expense. www.DrHoBelt.com. (877) 246-1117, (800) 801-5607.
7. **PHX True Pulse PEMF Device:** This therapy is based on pulsed electromagnetic field therapy. Electrical energy is used to send waves of magnetic pulses through the blood and tissue. Tiny electrical signals stimulate and massage the cells resulting in pain relief by relieving knots in the neck and back, and trigger point pain. www.pulsedharmonix.com.
8. **Low Level Lasers Q Laser System:** Low level lasers will reduce inflammation and pain. (800) 303-6923, code 7062.
9. **Elbow Knee Brace for Pain**: www.getcopperfit.com.

10. **Brace for Pain**: www.beactivebrace.com.
11. **VS 2 Versa Shock Sole:** This sole insert guards against harmful shock to joints resulting in 40 percent less harmful impact. Free trial for 30 days. www.gravitydefyer.com/MF9KDQ3. (800) 429-0039.
12. **Walk Fit:** Five million of these shoe inserts have been sold. They provide alignment to the body and give pain relief to feet, knees, and back. www.walkfitplatinum.com. (800) 606-4174.
13. **Good Feet Arch Supports:** These supports provide support for feet, knees, and back pain. www.goodfeettam-pabay.com.
14. **Grid STK Foam Roller:** The Grid STK Foam Roller is used for self-administered massage on painful areas of the body. A number of maladies are helped by the roller including age-related muscle tightness, muscle soreness from exercise, and tendinitis. Research shows it restores blood flow and disperses lactic acid. The Grid STK Foam Roller is sold at $34.99 and can be purchased at TPTherapy.com.
15. **Electronic Muscle Stimulator (EMS):** The EMS device delivers impulses through adhesive electrode pads, which relieves pain by addressing the root cause of most pain. The EMS units go well beyond disrupting the signal to relieve pain as a TENS unit. To order call (877) 317-2888, or go online to Hidowprofessional.com. The EMS device is registered with the FDA and the costs range from $150 to $350.
16. **Kyroback:** Kyroback is advertised as the only home-use device utilizing professional oscillation therapy and continuous passive motion. It has been clinically proven to treat lower back pain with lasting relief. A recent clinical study showed Kyroback provided three weeks of pain relief after usage was stopped. This home device is used just for ten minutes. The longer Kyroback users continued treatment, the more relief they reported. Kyroback can be used on the sofa, bed, and floor. There is a risk free trial for 60 days. Call (800) 971-1407 or go to www.kyrooffer271.com.

Eight Other Natural Pain Cures

1. **Leg Cramps** - A *bar of soap* in your bed will give off magnesium to relieve leg cramps.
2. **Burn Pain** - *Aloe vera* is an effective treatment for burns and abrasions.
3. **Insect Stings** - A *raw onion* is cooling and has enzymes that decrease inflammation.
4. **Head Pain** - A good *foot rub* can release pain-relieving endorphins.
5. **Ear Aches** - Warm *olive oil* may soothe ear pain temporarily and may loosen up wax that is causing pain.
6. **Toothache pain** - Rub *clove oil* into the gums to treat toothache.
7. **Gout** - *Cherries* have been linked to a 35 percent lower risk of gout attacks. Research has shown tart cherry juice reduces uric acid by 25 percent.
8. **Migraines** - A strong cup of *coffee* can ward off a migraine by constricting blood vessels in the brain. Caffeine also offsets the widening of blood vessels that occur during the migraine. Caffeine is listed on the labels of several pain killers including Excedrin and Anacin.

Appendix II

CHRONIC PAIN

Making A Decision About Pain Therapy
An Unorthodox Guide

After reading this book, you may be overwhelmed by the number of options for treating chronic pain. This appendix will provide guidance in making decisions regarding pain. It explains the principles involving the technique of applied kinesiology (muscle testing), and the pendulum (dowsing). These techniques are often used by alternative healers in providing guidance in choosing pain relief methods. It is based on quantum physics that shows that everything is interconnected, and there is no such thing as space and time. In other words, we are all one. This is explained in detail in my book *We Are One: The Science of Oneness*. All knowledge is available to everyone in the Universal Mind Matrix and can be tapped into with applied kinesiology and the pendulum. These disciplines transcend space and time. The Mind Matrix quantum field is all around us carrying information about the past, present, and future. By tapping into this subtle energy, we have the ability to be omniscient and all knowing. The knowledge of disease, including pain, is in the Universal Mind Matrix that can be tapped into. Other names for this quantum field is the collective conscious and implicate order as described by physicist David Bohm.

Applied Kinesiology

Muscle testing is a term used to describe applied kinesiology. Every muscle is connected to the health and pathology of a corresponding body organ. Muscles instantly become weaker when the body is exposed to a harmful stimulus and stronger when exposed to a therapeutic substance.

Muscle testing is a very simple technique. The subject extends one arm out straight to the side at shoulder height and is asked to provide resistance when the practitioner pushes the arm down. At some level below conceptual consciousness the body knows what is good or bad or true or false and that the knowing is registered in the muscles. The practitioner asks a 'yes' or 'no' question and then applies pressure to the extended arm. If the body's answer is 'no' or is harmful to the subject, the muscle becomes weak and the arm is easily pressed downward. If the answer is 'yes' or is beneficial to the subject, the arm remains firmly in place.

In the 1970s, John Diamond, M.D., refined muscle testing into a new discipline he called behavioral kinesiology. He taught his method to thousands of professionals around the world. His results were predictable, repeatable, and universal. Dr. Diamond found the body responded accurately, even when the conscious mind was unaware. For example, he found all classical music caused a universal strong response, and rock music produced a weak response.

Being able to test for truth intrigued David Hawkins, M.D., Ph.D., a renowned psychiatrist in New York City. In 1975, Hawkins began his kinesiology research in response to truth and falsehoods as described in his book *Power vs. Force*. Dr. Hawkins performed double blind tests in mass demonstrations. For example, he tested two substances concealed in identical envelopes. One envelope contained artificial sweeteners. The other held the placebo. He found that subjects tested weak in the envelope with the artificial sweetener and strong with the placebo. His research found that the questions had to be phrased so that the answer was clearly 'yes' or 'no.' Hawkins believed the brain is connected to a universal energy field. For twenty years, Hawkins analyzed the full spectrum of the level of human consciousness. He discovered that the anatomy consciousness produces a profile of the human condition. Hawkin's research found that the origin of emotional sickness lay in people's belief that they were their personalities. He found that nothing actually happens because past, present, and future are only artifacts of perception, as is the illusion of a 'separate' I that is subject to birth and death. Hawkins believed that it is only the illusion of individuality that is the origin of all suffering, which includes pain. When one realizes that he or she is one with the universe, there is no further suffering. Dr. Hawkins saw kinesiology as a 'wormhole' between two universes — the physical and the mind and spirit — an interface between dimensions.

Hawkins said "The individual human is like a computer terminal connected to a giant database. The data base is human consciousness with its roots in the common consciousness of all mankind. The unlimited information is contained in the database and now has been shown to be readily available to anyone in a few seconds at any time and place by kinesiology or dowsing." This includes the information about the cause and treatment of pain.

Hawkins' research revealed that the mind thinks with the body itself. The mind and body are one. Quantum physics has shown that the subjective and objective are one. If the subject and object are the same, time can be transcended. If they are one, then we can then find the answers merely by looking within man himself. The body can discern to the finest degree the difference between that which supports life and that which does not.

Dr. Hawkins' research method was used to verify the truth or falsehood of a declarative statement. He found that no reliable results could be obtained by inquiring into the future. Only statements regarding current or past events would produce consistent results. Kinesiology is now a well established science based on the testing of an all or none muscle response.

The Pendulum (Dowsing)

Dowsing is another technique to access the Universal Mind Matrix, often used for locating water for a well. The dowser asks the question with his mind and the two hand-held dowsing rods respond. When the dowser recognizes a movement in the rods or change in energy, the dowser identifies the location of water for a well.

Similar to the dowsing rod principle is the pendulum. The practitioner asks a 'yes' or 'no' question with his or her mind. A 'yes' response will cause the pendulum to swing in one direction and a 'no' response will cause the pendulum to move in the opposite direction. It can access the data bank of universal knowledge of everything that has happened in the universe which lies awaiting in the implicate order or Mind Matrix. Some practitioners can use the pendulum for dowsing percentages by asking a 'yes' or 'no' response.

Dowsing is an ancient practice that is still used today to find subsurface water and oil. The term 'water witching' is often used to describe the technique. Standard Oil, Getty Oil, and Rothschild Oil commonly used dowsers in the past to find oil. They also used it to find high volumes of water for oil refineries. Municipalities such as Flagstaff, Arizona have used dowsing to find water for the city. A number of studies have been conducted on dowsing and water exploration. One study in Sri Lanka found a 96 percent success rate of 691 wells drilled compared to a normal success rate of between 30 and 50 percent with traditional methods. Dowsing can also predict the depth of wells.

Researchers have found that it is not an electromagnetic energy but a psychic energy that produces the information of the dowsing rods or pendulum. Change in brain wave patterns in the dowser have been found and messages are registered in the subconscious and parasympathetic nervous system. Dowsers always ask 'yes' and 'no' questions. We all have the ability to be dowsers and applied kinesiologists to tap into the universal data base of knowledge.

Finding the Cause and Treatment of Chronic Pain

The reason for this chapter is to provide a starting point to determine the cause and treatment course for chronic pain. Listed are most of the chronic pain causes and treatments discussed in this book that can be tested by applied kinesiology or with the pendulum. The internet has a directory of those who are trained in applied kinesiology. You might check the yellow pages to see if any practitioners in your area use applied

Appendix II

kinesiology. Some chiropractors use applied kinesiology in their practice.

Greg Nielsen has written a number of books about the pendulum and is considered one of the top experts in this field. Greg is a university professor in Reno, Nevada in the Department of Education. He has the unique ability to provide a number value between one and ten for each question that gives the weight of a 'yes' or 'no' response. For example, he might get a reading of eight for the question about acupuncture being effective in treating your chronic pain. If the number four came up with another treatment, the treatment would not be as effective. Contact Greg at Greg.nielsen@charter.net. I want to emphasize these are only guidelines, a roadmap, in searching for the cause and treatment of your chronic pain. Once you have decided on a path of treatment, it would be prudent to check with your health care practitioner.

Name_____

Date_____ DOB_____

Address_____

Phone_____

(I) Causes of Chronic Pain
- A. Injury _____
- B. Mental/Emotional _____
- C. Repressed Emotion _____
- D. Diet _____
- E. Disease _____
- F. Sleep Disorder _____
- G. Lifestyle _____
- H. Allergy / Autoimmune _____
- I. Toxins _____
- J. Other _____

A. Mental/Emotional Causes
1. Hysteria _____
2. Hypochondria _____
3. Malingering _____
4. Post Traumatic Stress _____
5. Forgiveness Issues _____
6. Childhood Trauma _____
7. Mother Relationship _____
8. Father Relationship _____
9. No One to Love _____
10. Bereavement _____
11. Irritation _____
12. Isolation _____
13. Passivity _____
14. Masochism _____
15. Preoccupation with Pain _____
16. Resentment _____
17. Jealousy _____
18. Not Expressing Feelings _____
19. Not Loving Yourself _____
20. Not Sharing Pain Problem _____
21. Anger _____
22. Frustration _____
23. Helplessness _____
24. Hopelessness _____
25. Gain from Pain _____

Appendix II

26. Family Dynamics ____
27. Relationships ____
28. Anxiety ____
29. Depression ____
30. Confusion ____
31. Tension ____
32. Fear of Pain ____
33. Distress ____
34. Low Self Esteem ____
35. Stress ____
36. Sleep Disorder ____
37. Insomnia ____
38. Fear ____
39. Guilt ____
40. Not Understood ____
41. Why Me? ____
42. Feeling Unloved ____
43. Denial ____
44. Not Working ____
45. Fatigue ____
46. Worry ____
47. Financial Stress ____
48. Repressed Emotion ____
49. Mood Disorder ____
50. Panic Disorder ____
51. Obsessive Compulsive ____
52. Hyperalgesia ____
53. Other___

B. Diet

1. Food Allergies ____
2. Corn ____
3. Fast Food ____
4. Bread ____
5. Vegetable Oil ____
6. Corn Oil ____
7. Eggplant ____
8. Tomato ____
9. Potato ____
10. Dairy Products ____
11. Dietary Fat ____
12. Chocolate ____
13. Eggs ____
14. Citrus Food ____
15. Red Meat ____
16. Nuts ____
17. Onions ____
18. Apples ____
19. Bananas ____
20. Pasta ____
21. Nitrates in Food ____
22. Vitamin K Deficiency ____
23. Gluten ____
24. Caffeine ____
25. Calcium Deficiency ____
26. Monosodium Glutamide ____

27. Aspartamine ____
28. Refined Sugar ____
29. Vitamin D deficiency ____
30. Omega 6 Fatty Acids ____
31. Soft Drinks ____
32. Chemical Additives ____
33. Vitamin B12 Deficiency ____
34. Folic Acid Deficiency ____
35. Other ____

C. Lifestyle
1. Smoking ____
2. Alcohol ____
3. Lack of Creative Output ____
4. Not Found Life Purpose ____
5. Need a Pet ____
6. Environmental Toxins ____
7. Other ____

D. Health Causes
1. Ischemia ____
2. Osteoarthritis ____
3. Rheumatoid Arthritis ____
4. Women's Issues (Menopause, etc.) ____
5. Arachnoiditis ____
6. Fibromyalgia ____
7. Obesity ____
8. Gout ____
9. Cardiovascular Disease ____
10. Cancer ____
11. Diabetes ____
12. Trigeminal Neuralgia ____
13. Co-morbidity ____
14. Infectious Disease ____
15. Post Stroke Pain ____
16. Post Surgical Pain ____
17. Neuropathy ____
18. TMJ ____
19. Virus, Bacteria, Fungus ____
20. Low Blood Sugar ____
21. Back Disorder ____
22. Abnormal Muscle Fascia ____
23. Muscle Spasms ____
24. Spine Instability ____
25. Bulging Disk ____
26. Whiplash ____

Appendix II

27. Sciatica ____
28. Spinal Stenosis ____
29. Other ____

(II) Treatment of Chronic Pain

A. Prescription Drugs ____
B. Over the Counter Drugs ____
C. Surgery/Injections ____
D. Diet ____
E. Herbal Remedies ____
F. Vitamins/Minerals/Supplements ____
G. Exercise ____
H. Body Work ____
I. Energy/Subtle Energy Therapy ____
J. Stress Reduction/Forgiveness/Psychotherapy ____
K. Miscellaneous Therapies ____
L. Ayurvedic Medicine ____
M. Traditional Chinese Medicine ____
N. Amniotic Stem Cell Therapy ____
O. Spiritual ____
P. Lifestyle Change ____
Q. Other ____

A. Over-the-Counter Drugs

1. NSAID Drugs ____
2. Aspirin ____
3. Ibuprofen ____
4. Advil ____
5. Motrin ____
6. Nuprin ____
7. Profen ____
8. Excedrin ____
9. Acetaminophen ____
10. Tylenol ____
11. Topical NSAID ____
12. Topical Capsaicin (Axsaids) ____
13. Naproxen (Aleve) ____
14. Hyaluronanic Acid ____
15. Other ____

B. Prescription Drugs

1. Cox-2 Inhibitors ____
2. Celecoxib ____
3. Etodolal ____
4. Rofercoxib ____
5. Tricyclic Antidepressants ____
6. Desipramine ____

7. Amitriptyline ____
8. Amoxapine ____
9. Doxepin ____
10. Effexor ____
11. Duloxetine ____
12. Anticonvulsants ____
13. Gabapentin ____
14. Carbamazepine ____
15. Pregabaline ____
16. Amitrptyline ____
17. Cannabinoids ____
18. Esamet ____
19. THC Analog Nabilone ____
20. Marinol ____
21. Weak Opioids ____
22. Codeine ____
23. Dihydrocodeine ____
24. Dextropropoxphene ____
25. Strong Opioids ____
26. Morphine ____
27. Bupremorphine ____
28. Diamorphine (Heroin) ____
29. Fentanyl ____
30. Oxycodone ____
31. Percocet ____
32. Demerol ____
33. Valium ____
34. Xanax ____
35. Fiorinal ____
36. Zostrix ____
37. Klonopins ____
38. Elevil ____
39. Trazadone ____
40. Corticosteroids ____
41. Methionine ____
42. Diacerhein ____
43. Capsaicin ____
44. Carbamazepine ____
45. Oxcarbazepine ____
46. Lamotripran ____
47. Venla Faxine ____
48. S-Adenosylmethoine ____
49. IA Hyalurinic Acid ____
50. Lamotrigene ____
51. Zostric Cream ____
52. Topical Lidocaine ____
53. Other ____

C. **Diet**

1. Vegetarian Diet ____
2. Less Red Meat ____
3. Low Protein ____
4. High Complex Carbohydrate ____

Appendix II

5. Fruits and Vegetables _____
6. High Fiber _____
7. Fasting _____
8. Dong Diet _____
9. Fish Oil _____
10. Resveratrol _____
11. Fish _____
12. Eggs _____
13. Cheese _____
14. Polyunsaturated Fats _____
15. Beans _____
16. Fruit Juices _____
17. Green Tea _____
18. Herbal Tea _____
19. Mulberry Leaf Tea _____
20. Mint Tea _____
21. Hot Cinnamon Tea _____
22. Legumes _____
23. Tryptophan _____
24. Broccoli _____
25. Aloe Juice _____
26. Seaweed _____
27. Nuts _____
28. Licorice _____
29. Papaya _____
30. Prim Rose Oil _____
31. Cod Liver Oil _____
32. Gin Soaked Raisins _____
33. Avocados _____
34. Soybeans _____
35. Flaxseed Oil _____
36. Onions _____
37. Vegan Diet _____
38. Other _____

D. **Vitamins, Minerals, and Supplements**
1. Omega 3 Fatty Acids _____
2. Vitamin A _____
3. Vitamin C _____
4. Vitamin D _____
5. Vitamin E _____
6. B Vitamins _____
7. Vitamin B3 (Niacinamide) _____
8. Folate _____
9. Vitamin B5 (Pantothentic Acid) _____
10. Bioflavonoids _____
11. Magnesium _____
12. Zinc _____
13. Copper _____
14. Melatonin _____
15. Beta Carotene _____

16. Linolenic Acid ____
17. Shark Cartilage ____
18. Boron ____
19. Other ____

E. Herbs
1. Glucosamine ____
2. Chondroitin Sulfate ____
3. Rosehip ____
4. Harpagophytum Preparation ____
5. Ginger ____
6. Boswellia Serrata ____
7. Gum Resin ____
8. Willow Bark Abstract ____
9. Gingko Biloba ____
10. Ginger Bilberry ____
11. Dong Quai ____
12. Nettles ____
13. Hox Alpha ____
14. Rhus Toxicodendron Homeopathy ____
15. Cayenne Pepper ____
16. Capsamol Salve ____
17. Dolenon Liniment ____
18. St. John's Wort ____
19. Vitex ____
20. Agnolyt ____
21. Agnucaston ____
22. Cetanorm ____
23. Aloe Vera ____
24. Boswellia ____
25. Turmeric ____
26. Ashwaghanda ____
27. Bromelain ____
28. Chinese Herbs ____
29. Collagen Copper ____
30. Devil's Claw ____
31. DMSO ____
32. Echinacea ____
33. Gamma Gla ____
34. Ginseng ____
35. Guai Fenesin ____
36. Kava Kava ____
37. Methylsulfonylmethane (MSM) ____
38. Stinging Nettle ____
39. Thunder God Vine ____
40. Valerian Root ____
41. Comfrey Root ____
42. Chamomile ____
43. Kytta Plasmashia ____
44. Kitta Salve ____
45. Cramp Bark ____
46. Arnica ____
47. Tiger Balm ____

Appendix II

48. Guggol ____
49. Triphala ____
50. Skull Cap ____
51. Chrysanthemum Flower ____
52. White Flower ____
53. Shilajit ____
54. Black Bone Herb ____
55. Black Cherry ____
56. Goji Berries ____
57. Aclzuki Beans ____
58. Guto Kola ____
59. Common Butterbur ____
60. Pestilence Wort ____
61. Petadolex ____
62. Peppermint Oil ____
63. Chinese Peppermint ____
64. Euminz ____
65. Inspiral ____
66. Indian Frankincense ____
67. Achrathes ____
68. Gentiana ____
69. Licorice ____
70. Mallow ____
71. Cat's Claw ____
72. Other ____

F. **Herbal Remedies, Pills, and Oils**
1. Xiao Yao Wan ____
2. Ease 2 ____
3. Mobility 2 ____
4. Mobility 3 ____
5. Chinese Vine Essence ____
6. Avoca Asu ____
7. Triphala ____
8. Channel Flow ____
9. Three Immortal ____
10. Amla 25 ____
11. Agar 25 ____
12. Po Sumon Oil ____
13. Die Da Wan Hua Oil ____
14. Dit Da Jow ____
15. Kwan Loong Pain Relief ____
16. Oil of Eucalyptus ____
17. Other ____

G. **Exercise Therapy**
1. Dancing ____
2. Sex ____
3. Aqua Jogging ____
4. Strength Training ____
5. Gardening ____

6. Jogging _____
7. Hiking _____
8. Cycling _____
9. Stretching _____
10. Calisthenics _____
11. Aerobics _____
12. Golf _____
13. Skiing _____
14. Swimming _____
15. Yoga _____
16. Tai Chi _____
17. Gi Gong _____
18. Pilates _____
19. Weight Lifting _____
20. Other _____

H. Body Work Therapy
1. Massage _____
2. Reiki _____
3. Swedish Massage _____
4. Trigger Point Therapy _____
5. Physical Therapy _____
6. Occupational Therapy _____
7. Chiropractic _____
8. Osteopathy _____
9. Rolfing _____
10. Acupressure _____
11. Craniosacral Therapy _____
12. Kneading Therapy _____
13. Therapeutic Touch _____
14. Leech Therapy _____
15. Cupping _____
16. Moxibustion _____
17. Traction _____
18. Alexander Technique _____
19. Shiatsu _____
20. Canthaidan Plaster _____
21. Heat Therapy _____
22. Hot Tub _____
23. Sauna _____
24. Hot Water Bottle _____
25. Electric Heating Pad _____
26. Ice Packs _____
27. Ice Massage _____
28. Cold Spray _____
29. Other _____

I. Energy/Subtle Energy Therapy
1. Low Energy Laser _____
2. Magnet Therapy _____

Appendix II

3. Pulsed Electromagnetic Field ____
4. Crystal Therapy ____
5. Radionics ____
6. Gelsemium (Homeopathy) ____
7. Dulcanara (Homeopathy) ____
8. Arnica (Homeopathy) ____
9. LED Light ____
10. Biofeedback ____
11. TENS unit ____
12. High Frequency TENS ____
13. Low Frequency TENS ____
14. Acupuncture ____
15. Homeopathy ____
16. Kinesiology ____
17. Ayurvedic Medicine ____
18. Traditional Chinese Medicine ____
19. Laser Therapy ____
20. Ultrasound Therapy ____
21. Radio Frequency ____
22. Music Therapy ____
23. Ordnungs Therapy ____
24. Electroacupuncture ____
25. Laser Acupuncture ____
26. Electrotherapy ____
27. Magnetic Systems Machine ____
28. Naturopathy ____
29. Other ____

J. Mental/Stress Therapy

1. Develop Coping Skills ____
2. Visualization ____
3. Divert Attention ____
4. Cognitive Behavioral Therapy ____
5. Comfortable Environment ____
6. Hypnotherapy ____
7. Stress Management ____
8. Develop Positive Attitude ____
9. Breathing to Relax ____
10. Relaxation Tapes ____
11. Progressive Muscle Relaxation ____
12. Be Optimistic ____
13. Be Altruistic ____
14. Finding Life Purpose ____
15. Doing Life Purpose ____

16. Humor ____
17. Affirmations ____
18. Meditation ____
19. Prayer ____
20. Acknowledge Higher Power ____
21. Spirituality ____
22. Acknowledge and Release Repressed Emotion ____
23. Deep Relaxation ____
24. Psychotherapy ____
25. Develop Healthy Relationship____
26. Express Gratitude ____
27. Develop Sense of Purpose ____
28. Join Support Group ____
29. Emotion Freedom Technique ____
30. Laughter ____
31. Forgiveness____
32. Other ____

K. Miscellaneous Therapies

1. Semperflex (HSI) ____
2. Victoria (HSI) ____
3. Soothanol (HSI) ____
4. NT Factor (HSI) ____
5. Alpha Lipoic Acid Nerve Shield (HSI) ____
6. Blood of the Dragon (HSI) ____
7. Supple ____
8. Hyalgan Therapy ____
9. Prolozone Therapy ____
10. Feldenkraus Method ____
11. Emu Oil ____
12. Arthopure ____
13. Cold Laser Therapy ____
14. Copper Hands (Glove) ____
15. Eucalyptus Oil ____
16. Omega XL ____
17. Magna Life ____
18. Hydrolytic Enzymes ____
19. Yuen Method ____
20. Joint Flex ____
21. Platelet Rich Plasma Injection ____
22. Instaflex____
23. Pain Band (NGBalance.com) ____
24. Sun Chorella ____
25. Foot Reflexology ____
26. Gravity Defyer ____
27. Static Electricity ____

Appendix II

28. Prolo Therapy ____
29. Dog Therapy ____
30. Lighting for Pain ____
31. Anataflex ____
32. Soleve ____
33. Kyphoplasty ____
34. Denver Headache Center ____
35. Advanced Healthcare (Fort Collins, Injections)____
36. Neuropath Centers (Florida) ____
37. Placebo ____
38. Arthopure ____
39. Oxyrub ____
40. Instaflex ____
41. TENS____
42. Joint Flex____
43. Arthritis Relief Cream ____
44. Ostinol ____
45. Synerflex ____
46. Rezil ____
47. Painwizard ____
48. Nerve Shield ____
49. MagniLife Diabetic Neuropathy Foot Cream____
50. AloeCure ____
51. MagniLife Sciatica Relief ____
52. Triple Therapy Knee Pain Reliever ____
53. Frequency Band ____
54. Stem Cell Therapy ____
55. Dr. Ho's Decompression Belt ____
56. PHX True Pulse ____
57. Elbow Knee Brace ____
58. Low Level Lasers ____
59. Brace For Pain ____
60. Kyroback____
61. Sole Inserts ____
62. True Pulse A 2000____
63. Pain Pen____

REFERENCES AND SUGGESTED READING

Backer, Marcus and Hamme, Michael, *Acupuncture in the Treatment of Pain*, Elsevier, Edinburgh, 2010. Chapters 8, 9, 11, 12

Banks, Carol and Mackrodt, Karen, *Chronic Pain Management*, Whurr Publishers, London, 2001. Chapter 1, 3, 9, 12

Bond, Michael and Simpson, Karen, *Pain: Its Nature and Treatment*, Churchill Livingston (Elsevier), Edinburgh, 2006. Chapters 1, 2, 4, 8

Brownstein, Art, *Healing Back Pain Naturally*, Harbor Press, Inc, Gig Harbor, WA, 1999. Chapter 4

Centers for Disease Control, *Arthritis-Related Statistics*, 2014. Chapters 2, 3, 4, 11

Caudill, Margaret, *Managing Pain Before It Manages You*, The Guilford Press, New York, 1995. Chapters 1, 2, 3, 9, 10, 12

Chaitow, Leon, *Fibromyalgia Syndrome: A Practical Guide to Treatment*, Churchill Livingstone, Edinburgh, 2003. Chapter 7

Challem, Jack, *The Inflammation Syndrome*, John Wiley and Sons, Hoboken, NJ, 2003. Chapters 10, 11

Consumer Reports, *America's Scary Pain Pill Habit*, September 2014. Chapter 1

Consumers Report, *Deadly Pain Pills*, September 2014. Chapter 1, 6

Croft, Peter, Blyth, Fiona, and Vander Windt, Danielle, *Chronic Pain Epidemiology: From Etiology to Public Health*, Oxford University Press, Oxford, England, 2010. Chapters 1, 2, 3, 9, 10, 12

Elton, Diana, Stanley, Gordon, and Burrows, Graham, *Psychological Control of Pain*, Grune and Stratton, New York, 1983. Chapter 2

Ernst, Edzard, Pittler, May, and Wider, Barbara, *Complementary Therapies for Pain Management*, Elsevier Mosby, 2005. Chapters 2, 3, 4, 7, 8, 9, 11, 12

References and Suggested Reading

Fillingim, Roger, *Concise Encyclopedia of Pain Psychology*, The Haworth Medical Press, New York, 2005. Chapters 2, 3, 8

Foreman, Judy, *A Nation in Pain: Healing Our Biggest Health Problem*, Oxford University Press, New York, 2014. Preface

Gatchel, Robert and Turk, Dennis, *Psychological Approaches to Pain*, The Guilford Press, New York, 1996. Chapters 2, 3, 4, 8

Goldberg, Burton, *Alternative Medicine: The Definitive Guide*, Future Medicine Publishing, Inc, Puyallup, WA, 1993. Chapter 10

Hadady, Letha, *Naturally Pain Free*, Source Books, Naperville, IL, 2012. Chapters 4, 9, 11, 12

Horstman, Judith, *The Arthritis Foundation Guide to Alternative Therapies*, Arthritis Foundation, Atlanta, 1999. Chapters 2, 3, 6, 7, 9, 11, 12

Marcus, Dawn, *Chronic Pain: A Primary Care Guide*, Humana Press, Totowa, NJ, 2005. Chapters 2, 4, 7, 8, 10, 11

Null, Gary, *Reverse Arthritis and Pain Naturally: A Proven Approach to a Pain Free Life*, North Palm Beach, FL, 2013. Chapters 1, 2, 6, 9, 10, 11, 12

Prudden, Bonnie, *Pain Erasure: The Bonnie Prudden Way*, Ballantine Books, New York, 1980. Chapter 12

Rashig, Saifudin, et al, *Chronic Pain, A Healthy Perspective*, Wiley Blackwell, Germany, 2008. Chapters 1, 2, 3, 6, 7, 8

Sarno, John, *Mind Over Back Pain*, Berkley Books, New York, 1982. Chapter 5

Sarno, John, *Healing Back Pain: The Mind Body Connection*, Warner Books, New York, 1991. Chapter 5

Sarno, John, *The Mind Body Prescription*, Warren Books, New York, 1998. Chapter 5

Stahl, Stephen, *Chronic Pain and Fibromyalgia*, Cambridge University Press, 2009. Chapters 1, 2, 7

Staugaard-Jones, Jo Ann, *Back Pain Mystery Solved*, Bottom/Line Health, November 2015. Chapter 4

Thacker, Emily, *Vinegar Anniversary Book*, James Direct Inc., Hartsville, OH, 2006. Chapter 6

Theodosakis, Jason, *The Arthritis Cure*, Affinity Communications Corp, New York, 1999. Chapters 6, 11

The Prevention Pain Relief System, Editors of *Prevention Magazine*, Health Books, Rodale Press, Emmaus, PA, 1992. Chapters 2, 3, 4, 8, 9, 10, 11, 12

Vad, Vijay, *Arthritis RX*, Gotham Books, New York, 2006. Chapters 6, 10, 11

Wright, Jonathan, *Treasury of Natural Cures*, New Market Publishing, Baltimore, 2013. Chapter 10

Index

A

Acceptance 40
Acetaminophen 7, 235
Acid Reflux 144
Acupressure 58, 137, 193, 240
Acupuncture 79, 110, 124, 125, 131, 135, 143, 146, 149, 191-193, 202, 204, 214, 215, 231, 241, 244
Adenosine 12, 14
Aerobics 48, 240
Affirmations 37, 242
Agar 35 150, 168
Alcohol 95, 97, 130, 148, 157, 164, 166, 234
Alexander, Franz 80
Alexander Technique 193, 194, 240
Allergies 16, 17, 62, 67, 70, 74, 106, 108, 109, 110, 112, 132, 144, 151, 154, 155, 159, 160, 163, 165, 166, 195, 233
Aloe Vera 102, 144, 168, 238
Alphalipoic Acid 142
Alzheimer's Disease 14, 15, 151, 156, 163, 181, 185, 212
American College of Rheumatology 105, 171
Ames, Bruce 162
Amitriptyline 122, 236
Amla 25 150, 169, 239
Andrographic 149
Anger 2, 20, 23, 25-27, 37, 66, 70-74, 79, 134, 199, 232
Ankylosing Spondylitis 95, 188
Antibiotic 9, 57
Antidepressants 119, 121, 122, 141, 235
Anxiety 1, 2, 11, 19, 21-25, 27, 29-35, 37, 39, 44, 46, 49, 66, 67, 70-74, 77, 79, 106, 108, 113, 115, 116, 120, 122, 124, 126, 133, 145, 147-150, 156, 157, 168, 178, 194, 199, 201, 202, 204, 210, 211, 233

Applied Kinesiology 218, 227-231
Aqua Therapy 93
Arachidonic Acid 96, 153, 155, 164
Arginine 124
Arnica 51, 55, 145, 168, 222, 238, 241
Aroma Therapy 146, 194
Arthopure 219, 242, 243
Arthritis iii, 1, 4, 5, 8, 12-16, 21, 26, 31, 33, 38, 41, 45, 53, 65, 81-89, 91-105, 111, 116, 123, 125, 143, 151, 152, 154-157, 159-165, 168-171, 173-180, 182-189, 193, 195-198, 200-203, 205, 208, 210-213, 215, 216, 219-222, 224, 234, 243, 244, 245
Arthritis Foundation 175, 185, 245
Ashwaganda 169, 170
Aspartame 125, 166
Aspirin 1, 7, 12, 53, 85, 90, 94, 102, 161, 167, 170, 171, 176-178, 180, 181, 184, 235
Asthma 16, 32, 34, 67, 70, 85, 151, 154, 170, 196, 204
Attitude 35-39, 52, 90, 199, 241
Autogenic Training 34
Avocado 169
Ayurvedic Medicine 57, 102, 169, 178, 182, 183, 194, 195, 235, 241

B

Back Pain iii, 1, 3, 4, 13, 19, 22, 24, 27, 32-34, 38, 41-55, 57, 59, 60-73, 75-77, 79, 104, 150, 161, 168, 172-174, 177, 178, 180, 182, 183, 193, 194, 196, 198, 200-204, 206, 211, 212, 215, 216, 218, 221, 224, 225, 244, 245
Balneotherapy 126, 200, 215
Barnes, Broda 120
Baron, Jill 21
Bee Sting Therapy 195
Beta Carotene 122, 149, 185, 237
Big Pharma 2, 6, 8

Biking 135
Biofeedback 29, 31, 32, 123, 131, 133, 135, 138, 210, 241
Biotin 142
Bisphenol-A 156
Black Cherry 149, 169, 239
Body Mass Index 155
Bohm, David 227
Bone Spur 45, 54, 65, 83
Boron 51, 101, 179, 188, 189, 220, 238
Boswellia 102, 169, 170, 219-221, 238
Bradykinin 12
Breathing 32-34, 40, 47, 49, 67, 91, 116, 135, 147, 200, 209, 241
Bromelain 51, 90, 99, 100, 167, 170, 187, 238
Brownstein, Art 19, 20, 38, 40, 45-49, 52, 53, 244
Butterbur 132, 170, 239

C

Caffeine 50, 97, 129, 132, 164, 166, 226, 233
Calcium 14, 57, 87, 88, 101, 108, 121, 124, 188, 189, 233
Calisthenics 48, 240
Cancer ii-vi, 8, 9, 13-15, 17, 20, 33, 37, 87, 104, 111, 146, 147, 149, 151, 152, 154-156, 160, 162, 163, 170, 171, 177, 181-183, 189, 193, 195, 196, 206, 207, 209, 210, 212, 216, 234
Candida 123, 144
Cannaboid / Cannabis 147, 171, 195
Cantharidin Plaster 196
Capsaicin 102, 142, 171, 222, 235, 236
Carbamazepine 141, 236
Carotenoids 16, 158
Carpal Tunnel Syndrome 75
Cartilage 53, 83-85, 87-90, 92, 98, 100, 101, 103, 123, 143, 161, 163, 164, 172, 176, 181, 182, 186, 187, 208, 209, 211, 220, 238
Cat's Claw 102, 172, 239
Caudill, Margaret 21-23, 244
Cayenne 97, 102, 158, 165, 171, 181, 238
Cayenne Red Pepper 171
Celebrex 86, 181, 221
Celecoxib 85, 235
Center for Disease Control 5, 92, 105
Cerebral Cortex 12
Chaitow, Leon 105, 120
Challem, Jack 15, 16, 157, 244
Chamomile 50, 58, 172, 238

Channel Flow 149, 150, 239
Chemotherapy Pain 140
Cherries 95, 98, 226
Childers, Norman 165
Childhood Abuse 26
Chiropractor 59, 60, 63, 65, 119, 196, 197, 224, 231
Chondroitin 88, 89, 100, 163, 172, 238
Chopra, Deepak 194
Chronic Fatigue 25, 74, 76, 106, 112, 114-118, 150, 210
Cluster Headaches 3, 137, 138
Coen, Stanley 76
Co-Enzyme Q 10 133
Cognitive Behavioral Therapy 35, 143, 241
Cold Packs 59, 215
Colitis 62, 67, 170, 221
Collagen 84, 88, 89, 101, 164, 173, 175, 176, 186, 220, 238
Comfrey 50, 102, 173, 238
Coping 22, 29, 35, 36, 39, 41, 44, 59, 70, 115, 198, 213, 241
Copper 101, 188, 197, 224, 237, 238, 242
Copper Bracelet 197
Cordain, Loren 159
Cortisol 13, 21, 22, 107, 117
Cousins, Norman 38
Crampbark 50, 150, 173
Cranial Electrotherapy 136
Cranial Sacral Therapy 197
C Reactive Protein 15, 17, 152, 153, 159-161, 163, 164
Crepitus 84
Crohn's Disease 162, 170, 221
Cupping 197, 214, 240
Cycling 48, 93, 240
Cyclooxygenase 85, 86

D

Dairy 96, 97, 110, 153, 155, 159, 160, 164, 165, 185, 233
Decursinol 100
Dental Amalgams 154
Depression 1, 2, 4, 8, 11, 19, 22-24, 26, 30, 37, 39, 44, 51, 72-74, 79, 82, 91, 106, 108, 111, 112, 114-116, 122, 124, 130, 133, 149, 150, 156, 174, 181, 182, 197, 199, 202, 203, 210, 211, 233
Devil's Claw 102, 174, 238
DHEA 174
Diabetes v, vi, 15, 17, 140, 141, 149, 150, 152, 154, 155, 156, 160, 163, 179, 183, 234

Index

Diabetic Neuropathy 12, 104, 140, 141, 142, 143, 171, 180, 212, 216, 223, 243
Diamond, John 228
Digestive Disorders 70, 71
Dit Da Jow 146, 239
DMSO 175, 179, 238
Dopamine 157, 181
Dorsal Root Ganglion 11
Dowsing 218, 227, 229, 230
Dulcamara 174

E

Electroacupuncture 125, 241
Emotions 2, 11, 19-21, 26, 28, 47, 52, 53, 60, 63, 67, 69-72, 76, 78-80, 109, 115, 143, 201, 214
Encephalins 38, 46, 52, 192
Endorphins 14, 38, 46, 52, 108, 122, 124, 134, 135, 157, 171, 192, 224, 226
Engel, George 20, 26
Enkephalin 14
Epileptic 32, 119
Epinephrine 21
Epstein-Barr Virus 74
Ergo Mania 28
Estrogen 87, 156, 160, 174
Exercise 5, 38, 39, 46, 48, 53-56, 59, 67, 79, 84, 86, 87, 91-95, 118, 121, 124, 126, 134, 135, 146, 152, 156, 157, 191, 195, 198, 200, 205, 206, 207, 209, 213, 214, 223, 225, 235, 239

F

Fasting 95, 198, 237
Fatigue iii, 11, 21, 25, 74, 76, 93, 104-108, 110, 112, 114-118, 122, 124, 127, 130, 146, 150, 168, 169, 174, 188, 201, 210, 233
Fear 6, 20, 38, 40, 46-48, 52, 63, 67, 71, 73, 77, 78, 115, 233
Federal Drug Agency 6
Feldenkrause Technique 199
Fenoprofen 85
Fever Few 175
Fiber 12, 50, 144, 159, 203, 237
Fibromyalgia iii, 1, 3, 19, 22-26, 31, 34, 39, 70, 74-76, 82, 92, 104-127, 177-179, 181, 184, 188, 193, 198, 200, 201, 203, 206, 209, 212, 223, 234, 244, 245
Fillingim, Roger 36
Flavonoids 16, 158, 160
Forgiveness 37, 39, 199, 232, 235, 242

Free Radicals 16, 96, 154, 155
Freud, Sigmund 20, 79
Frieden, Thomas 7
Fruits 16, 57, 96-98, 143, 152, 155, 158, 165, 179, 181, 183, 189, 237

G

Gabapentin 119, 141, 236
Gamma Linolenic Acid 101, 149, 162, 186
Garlic 96, 100, 148, 154, 158, 167
Gastrointestinal Bleeding 85
Gatchel, Robert 27, 28, 41
Gate Theory 14
Gi Gong 240
Ginger 100, 102, 144, 165, 167, 170, 175-177, 181, 183, 220, 222, 238
Gingko Biloba 146, 238
Ginseng 102, 148, 167, 169, 238
Gin-Soaked Raisins 175
Glucosamine 88-90, 101, 102, 163, 164, 176, 177, 186, 219, 220, 238
Glutathione 96, 101, 117, 154, 187
Gluten 17, 97, 106, 110, 125, 144, 159, 160, 233
Glycosaminoglycans 88, 163
Goji Berries 149, 239
Goldberg, Burton 57
Gout 3, 81, 82, 84, 95-97, 149, 152, 169, 188, 221, 226, 234
Grape Seed Extract 101, 177, 186, 220
Grape Seed Oil 97, 159, 165
Green Tea 100, 160, 165, 177, 186, 237
Group Therapy 41, 123
Growth Hormone 13, 22, 108, 116, 117, 124
Guafemesia 177
Guaifenesin 126
Guan Jie Yan Wan 177
Guggal 178
Guided Imagery 32, 199
Guilt 20, 27, 47, 66, 71, 233

H

Hadady, Letha 57, 149
Hawkins, David 228, 229
Headaches iii, v, 1, 3, 24, 26, 31-34, 62, 67, 70, 71, 73, 76, 111, 112, 129-138, 166, 171, 175, 178, 180, 183, 184, 193-198, 201, 205, 206, 210, 221, 222
Heart Attack 13, 15, 86, 161

Helplessness 37, 232
Herniated Disc 56, 64, 221
Hip 56, 81, 83, 86, 87, 169, 216
Honey 97, 100, 165, 182, 221
Horse Chestnut 178
Hot Packs 59
Humor 37, 38, 52, 242
Hyaluronic Acid 101, 219
Hydrocodon 7
Hydrotherapy 58, 126, 200
Hylan 86
Hyperventilation 109, 116
Hypnosis 29, 40, 41, 131, 136, 148, 201
Hypoglycemia 70, 121
Hypothyroidism 108, 120

I

Ibuprofen 1, 7, 12, 53, 55, 85, 88, 89, 161, 177, 221, 235
Imagination 33, 131, 199
Indigestion 143, 144, 168, 172
Inflammation 5, 12, 14-17, 21, 22, 32, 49, 51, 53, 55, 57, 59, 66, 83, 84, 86, 91, 95, 96, 97-101, 107, 126, 138, 146, 150-155, 157, 160-166, 168, 170, 172-175, 177-179, 183, 184-187, 192, 201, 203, 204, 222, 224, 226, 244
Insomnia 1, 11, 24, 25, 32, 34, 116, 150, 172, 178, 194, 233
Institute of Medicine iv, 8
Insulin Resistance 17, 95, 163
Irritable Bowel Syndrome 107, 111, 113, 143, 145, 180, 193, 196, 201, 210

J

Jogging 46, 48, 78, 94, 239, 240

K

Kesche Foundation, 217, 218
Knee 6, 36, 55, 56, 81-83, 86-89, 93, 103, 169, 176, 177, 187, 193, 198, 202, 203, 208, 209, 212, 215, 216, 219, 221, 224, 243
Knee Replacement 6, 83, 86

L

Laser Therapy 126, 131, 201, 202, 221, 241, 242
Lazer, Alan 208

Leape, Lucian L. 6
Lectin 125, 159
Leech Therapy 202, 240
Leukotrines 12, 176, 221
Light Emission Diode (LED) iv, 202, 224
Limbic System 11, 12, 67, 131, 194
Linoleic Acid 153, 154
Linolenic Acid 101, 153, 162, 186, 238
Loeser, John 75
Love 39, 52, 131, 232
Low Back Pain 27, 41, 43-45, 53, 54, 64, 75, 161, 174, 178, 180, 193, 201, 203, 204, 206, 215
L-tryptophan 124, 148, 149
Lupus 81, 92, 174, 210
Lutein 158
Lycopine 158
Lyme disease 76, 115

M

Macular Degeneration 104, 212
Magnesium 51, 57, 101, 113, 121, 124, 130, 148, 160, 177, 188, 189, 226, 237
Magnets 57, 126, 146, 203, 204
Malic Acid 124
Marcus, Dawn 59, 119, 120, 245
Marijuana 126, 147, 171, 195, 196
Massage 43, 55, 58, 79, 122, 134, 136, 145, 146, 194, 195, 197, 202, 203, 207, 210, 215, 224, 225, 240
McRae, Donald 64
Meditation 32, 39-41, 47, 49, 91, 92, 126, 133, 200, 204, 206, 209, 210, 242
Mediterranean Diet 161, 162, 164
Melatonin 51, 127, 179, 237
Memory 106, 108, 112, 115, 118, 171, 196
Mercury 117, 154, 157
Methyl Sulfonyl Methane 238
Migraine 32, 62, 67, 129-134, 170, 175, 178, 192, 198, 210, 226
Mobility 2 58, 239
Monosodium Glutamate 130, 166
Morphine 30, 38, 46, 236
Moxibustion 204, 214, 240
MSM 101, 179, 187, 220, 238
Mulberry Leaf Tea 179, 237
Multiple Sclerosis 104, 140, 152, 171, 199, 212
Muscle Relaxation 32, 34, 241
Muscle Spasm 14, 46, 50, 53, 59, 62, 193, 208, 234

Index

Muscle Testing 218, 227, 228
Musculoskeletal Pain 3, 170, 180, 181, 194, 196
Myofascitis 70

N

N-acetylcysteine 16
Naloxone 30
National Institute of Health v, vii, 6
National Institute of Mental Health 21
Naturopath 51, 105, 205, 241
Nerve Fiber 12
Nettles 102, 179, 180, 238
Neuropathy iii, 12, 104, 139-143, 145, 171, 180, 193, 198, 203, 204, 212, 216, 221, 223, 234, 243
Niacinamide 101, 186, 237
Nitric Oxide 12, 114, 117, 163
Nociception 10-13
NSAIDs 12, 85, 86, 94, 120, 141, 161, 169, 172, 180, 181, 185, 188, 207, 219, 235
Null, Gary 4-10, 95, 100, 152, 155, 156, 164, 168, 184-188, 245

O

Obesity 8, 17, 44, 82, 87, 93, 95, 129, 152, 155, 156, 183, 234
Olive Oil 97, 158, 161, 162, 164, 165, 222, 226
Omega 3 Fatty Acids 96, 100, 101, 153, 154, 157-162, 186, 237
Omega 6 Fatty Acids 96, 153, 154, 159, 160, 162, 234
Omega 9 Fatty Acids 158, 159, 161, 162
Opioid 7, 122, 192, 204, 236
Optimism 37, 38
Ordnungs Therapy 206, 207, 241
Oregano 158, 181, 222
Organic 97, 155, 160, 165
Osteoarthritis 3, 17, 23, 34, 36, 41, 81-93, 96, 98, 102, 104, 151, 152, 160-165, 169, 171, 172, 175-177, 179-181, 183, 185, 189, 193, 194, 196, 198, 200-205, 208, 209, 212-218, 220-222, 234
Osteopath 105, 197, 206, 240
Oxycodone 142, 236
Oxytocin 192

P

Pain Pen / Pain Pad 217, 243

Pain Receptors 11, 13, 46
Parkinson's Disease 104, 212
Passion Flower 51
Peale, Norman Vincent 37
PEMF 208, 209, 224
Peppermint Oil 136, 239
Phantom Limb 12, 19, 28, 41, 147
Physiatry 206
Physical Abuse 26, 114, 145
Physical Therapists 207
Physical Therapy 31, 59, 78, 79, 118, 119, 123, 207, 240
Phytodolor 180
Phytotherapy 207
Pilates 55, 91, 93, 240
Pinched Nerve 45, 46, 62, 65
Placebo 2, 6, 19, 29, 30, 40, 77, 89, 90, 119, 120, 131, 132, 135, 136, 145, 148, 162, 163, 169, 170, 173, 174, 176, 180, 183, 185, 189, 197, 202-204, 209, 211, 228, 243
Platelet Rich Plasma (PRP) 104, 207, 212, 242
PMS 110, 148, 149, 180, 183, 193, 203, 209
Post Herpetic Neuralgia 140, 141
Posturology 208
Prayer 29, 38, 52, 211, 242
Primrose Oil 142
Probiotics 187
Propranolol 121
Prostaglandin 12, 101, 153, 154, 161, 172, 176, 183, 186
Proteoglycans 84, 88, 89, 163, 176
Prozac 122
PRP 207, 208
Pulsed Electromagnetic Field (PEMF) 208, 209, 216, 224, 241

Q

Qigong 39, 92, 93, 198, 206, 209
Quercetin 101, 158, 187

R

Raynaud's Disease 22, 31
Red Clover 181
Referred Pain 13
Refined Foods 57, 86, 96, 97, 152, 156, 159, 164, 228, 234
Reflexology 147, 203, 209, 210, 242
Reiki 203, 210, 240
Relaxation Technique 49, 136, 204

Repetitive Stress 75, 76
Repressed Emotions 2, 19, 21, 28, 53, 60, 69, 70, 71
Resinall E 181
Rheumatoid Arthritis 12, 31, 41, 81, 82, 86, 91-104, 116, 125, 151, 152, 157-165, 170-180, 183-189, 198, 200-203, 210-216, 221, 234
Rhus Tox 58
Rhus Toxicodendron 200, 238
Rolfing 210, 240
Rosomoft, H. L. 64

S

Sacroiliac Pain 54
S-adenosyl-L-methionine 101, 124, 181, 187, 236
Salicylates 180-182
SAM-e 181, 187
Sarno, John 60-80
Schraeder, Harold 76
Sciatica 56-58, 64, 223, 235, 243
Scoliosis 45, 65
Sedimentation Rate 15, 164
Selenium 51, 101, 124, 157, 188
Self Efficacy 36
Serotonin 13, 14, 107, 108, 117, 119, 132, 148, 157, 181, 182, 192
Sexual Abuse 20, 26, 71, 114, 145
Seyle, Hans 21
Shark Cartilage 182, 238
Shiatsu 203, 210, 211, 240
Shilajit 182, 239
Shoulder 56, 62, 63, 65, 66, 68-70, 75, 83, 84, 134, 193, 199, 203, 209, 211, 228
Siegal, Bernie 20
Skiing 240
Sleep 7, 21, 23-25, 31, 50, 51, 57, 74, 93, 107, 108, 111-118, 120, 124-127, 149, 152, 169, 179, 183, 184, 223, 224, 232, 233
Smith, Melissa Diane 159
Spina Bifida 65
Spirituality 38, 52, 242
Spondylitis 65, 95, 188
Spondylolisthesis 56
Stahl, Stephen 106
Staugaard-Jones, Jo Ann 54, 245
Stem Cell 103, 104, 123, 143, 208, 211, 212, 220, 235, 243
Stenosis 54, 56, 235
St. John's Wort 51, 58, 148, 182, 222, 238

Stossel, John 61
Stress 1, 2, 11, 13, 16, 19-23, 30-35, 40, 44-47, 49, 53, 60-69, 72-76, 96, 98, 99, 100, 107, 110, 114-117, 129, 130, 133, 134, 138, 145, 150, 152, 154, 157, 168, 169, 194, 198-205, 210, 217, 232, 233, 235, 241
Stretching 47, 48, 53, 56, 92, 203, 207, 240
Strokes 86, 87
Substance P 13, 14, 108, 110, 117, 171
Suicide v, 4, 47
Superoxide Dismutase 101, 187
Support Groups 213
Surgery 1-6, 10, 24, 47, 54, 66, 75, 84, 87, 92, 94, 118, 147, 148, 181, 207, 208, 216, 235
Swimming 46, 48, 93, 135, 240
Synovial Fluid 83, 85
Szasz, Thomas 20

T

Tai Chi 92, 93, 198, 213, 240
TCM 213, 214
Telaxation Technique 29, 31, 34, 40, 47, 198, 200, 210
Temporal Mandibular Disorders 3, 32, 183, 197
TENS 58, 131, 135, 136, 215, 216, 224, 225, 241, 243
Tension Headaches 33, 67, 129, 133-136, 180, 210
Tension Myositis Syndrome (TMS) 63-80
Thalamus 11, 116, 117
THC 171, 196, 236
Theodosakis, Jason 84
Therapeutic Touch 135, 203, 214, 240
Thermal Therapy 215
Thiamine 57, 123
Three Immortal 150, 174, 239
Thromboxane 161, 164
Thunder God Vine 182, 238
Thyroid 13, 104, 108, 110, 113, 120, 121, 212
Thyroid Hormone 121
Tiger Balm 51, 136, 183, 238
Tiznidine 120
Traditional Chinese Medicine (TCM) 92, 149, 183, 213, 214, 235, 241
Trans-Fatty Acids 154
Trauma 15, 20, 23, 26, 27, 48, 57, 71, 83, 84, 85, 87, 107, 109, 111, 118, 145, 214, 221, 232
Tricyclic Antidepressants 119, 121, 141, 235

Index

Trigeminal Neuralgia 12, 140, 141, 193, 234
Trigger Points 110, 121, 192, 205
Trigger Point Therapy 203, 240
Triphala 58, 183, 239
True Pulse A 2000 216, 217, 243
Turmeric 57, 102, 165, 170, 181, 183, 219, 220, 222, 223, 238
Type 2 Diabetes 141
Type "A" 66, 72
Tyramine 130

U

Ulcers 15, 62, 71, 75, 76, 85, 144, 168, 188
Ultrasound 207, 217, 241
Uric Acid 95, 97, 178, 226

V

Vad, Vijay 33, 83, 86, 165
Valerian 25, 50, 126, 148, 184, 238
Valium 78, 236
Vegan 95-97, 125, 164, 237
Vegetarian 96, 155, 158, 164, 198
Vicodin 7, 8
Vinegar 100, 136, 182, 221, 245
Vioxx 86
Visualization 29, 31, 40, 47, 49, 133, 199, 200, 241
Vitamin A 98, 149, 185, 237
Vitamin B 51, 101, 121, 186
Vitamin B1 57, 186
Vitamin B3 186, 237
Vitamin B5 186
Vitamin B6 130, 142, 146, 148, 186
Vitamin B12 57, 142, 181, 234
Vitamin C 16, 51, 98, 110, 121, 158, 163, 164, 177, 185-187, 237
Vitamin D 87, 88, 142, 185, 234, 237
Vitamin E 16, 51, 57, 101, 122, 124, 130, 148, 158, 162, 163, 167, 185, 187, 237
Vitamin K 97, 98, 101, 181, 187, 233

W

Walking 48, 93, 134, 135
Weight Lifting 46, 48, 198, 240
Whiplash 76, 109, 234
White Flower 183, 239
Willow Bark 51, 58, 102, 184, 219, 238
Work 1, 4, 8, 10, 20, 27-29, 34, 43, 44, 47, 52, 55, 59, 61, 62, 66, 70, 75, 77, 78, 80, 82, 91, 94, 119, 122, 130, 138, 141, 142, 152, 185, 203, 206, 221
Wright, Jonathan 148, 165

X

Xiau Yao Wan 149

Y

Yoga 46, 48, 49, 55, 56, 91-93, 133, 136, 145, 198, 206, 217, 218, 240
Yucca 184
Yunnan Paiyao 184

Z

Zinc Sulfate 189
Zingerflex 102
Zylka, Mark v

CPSIA information can be obtained
at www.ICGtesting.com
Printed in the USA
FSOW01n0326160816
23731FS